HITLER'S
MALADIES

AND THEIR IMPACT ON WORLD WAR II

HITLER'S MALADIES

AND THEIR IMPACT ON WORLD WAR II

A BEHAVIORAL NEUROLOGIST'S VIEW

TOM HUTTON MD, PHD

TEXAS TECH UNIVERSITY PRESS

This book is typeset in EB Garamond. The paper used in this book meets the minimum requirements of ANSI/NISO Z39.48-1992 (R1997). ♾

Designed by Hannah Gaskamp; cover photograph by Shawshots / Alamy Stock Photo

Library of Congress Cataloging-in-Publication Data

Names: Hutton, J. Thomas, author. Title: Hitler's Maladies and Their Impact on World War II: A Behavioral Neurologist's View / Tom Hutton MD, PhD. Description: Lubbock, Texas: Texas Tech University Press, [2023] | Includes bibliographical references and index. | Summary: "A neurobehavioral analysis of Adolf Hitler drawn from a lifetime of medical research and clinical experience"—Provided by publisher.
Identifiers: LCCN 2022041352 (print) | LCCN 2022041353 (ebook)
ISBN 978-1-68283-166-3 (paperback) | ISBN 978-1-68283-167-0 (ebook)
Subjects: LCSH: Hitler, Adolf, 1889–1945—Health. | Hitler, Adolf, 1889–1945—Mental health. | Hitler, Adolf, 1889–1945—Military leadership. | Parkinson's disease—Patients—Germany—Biography. | Heads of state—Germany—Biography. | World War, 1939–1945—Germany. Classification: LCC DD247.H5 H888 2023 (print) | LCC DD247.H5 (ebook)
DDC 943.086092 [B]—dc23/eng/20220902
LC record available at https://lccn.loc.gov/2022041352
LC ebook record available at https://lccn.loc.gov/2022041353

Printed in the United States of America
23 24 25 26 27 28 29 30 31 / 9 8 7 6 5 4 3 2 1

Texas Tech University Press
Box 41037
Lubbock, Texas 79409-1037 USA
800.832.4042
ttup@ttu.edu
www.ttupress.org

Appreciation is due to those who fought and sacrificed during World War II and stemmed the rising surge of authoritarianism and Nazism. It is with great respect that we acknowledge those men and women who gave their todays so that we could enjoy the freedom of our tomorrows. Let us never forget those who mobilized for war and to whom the American newscaster, Tom Brokaw, referred as "the greatest generation." To this marvelous generation, whose numbers are now largely depleted, this book is dedicated.

CONTENTS

ILLUSTRATIONS

CHRONOLOGY OF ADOLF HITLER'S HEALTH AND SOCIAL / POLITICAL / MILITARY STATUS

	Physical / Mental Health	Social / Political / Military Status
April 20, 1889	Adolf Hitler born Braunau am Inn, Austria.	Father, a fifty-two-year-old doctrinaire Austrian customs official; mother, twenty-nine-year-old poorly educated, loving, hardworking woman.
1889–1903	Routine colds and flu for Adolf, but four of his five full siblings die of infectious diseases. Harsh emotional and physical abuse and humiliation by father.	Adolf poor student in Realschule; showed poor conduct, stubbornness, acting out; left school without graduating.
1903	Good physical health, routine viral illnesses, but psychologically terrorized by schizophrenic, deformed aunt. A loner.	Alcoholic father Alois Sr. dies.
1907	Good physical health, routine viral illnesses. Hitler claimed an uncorroborated pulmonary illness. Depression results from his failures in Vienna and deep grief over his mother's death.	Fails admission to Vienna Academy of Fine Arts. Unable to apply to architecture school due to lack of preparation and lack of graduation from Realschule. Mother Klara dies.
1907–1913	Good physical health but personality traits harden. Alleged exposure to syphilis by Viennese prostitute.	Menial jobs in Vienna, relative deprivation. Adrift and purposeless. Develops strident anti-Semitism and nationalistic views.
1914–1918	Shrapnel leg wounds and later gassed in mustard gas attack with transient visual loss. Germany's defeat in WWI prompts second loss of vision (hysterical visual loss).	Serves in German Army during World War I as courier. Lectures fellow troops; prudish and unpopular with comrades, yet brave under combat conditions, winning Iron Cross.
1919	Enjoys reasonably good health other than lifelong gastrointestinal (GI) complaints.	Serves in Munich in postwar German Army and spies for Weimar Republic on suspect political groups.
1919	Enjoys reasonably good health other than GI complaints and develops hoarseness.	Quits job for government; joins German Workers' Party, a nationalistic, anti-Semitic party that grows dramatically under Hitler's leadership and oratory.
1923	Sustains broken scapula in failed Beer Hall Putsch.	Convicted of treason and lands in Landsberg prison where he writes *Mein Kampf.*

1929	Increase in bloating sensation, constipation, and prominent flatulence during great stress (likely irritable bowel syndrome). Becomes vegetarian.	Worldwide depression and war reparations hit Germany particularly hard.
1932	Bothered by symptoms of IBS and hoarseness.	Loses run for German presidency to Paul von Hindenburg.
1933–1934	Stops swinging left arm when walking and handwriting becomes increasingly micrographic (signs of Parkinson's disease).	Appointed Reich Chancellor by President Hindenburg. Purges enemies in Nazi Party and bans other political parties.
1936	Develops chest tightening on exertion, coronary artery disease (CAD), with preceding moderate high blood pressure.	Sends troops into Rhineland and shares plans for territorial expansion and preparation for war.
1941	Angina pectoris attack during argument with von Ribbentrop and worsening heart complaints. Prostrating dysentery in August and probable gall bladder attack in September. PD worsens. Morell belatedly documents tremor.	Invasion of Russia, June 1941. German conquest of Yugoslavia and Greece. Addition of Moscow as strategic target to Operation Barbarossa proceeds lacking Hitler's presence; an overextension of German troops results in major military strategic error.
1943	Advancing heart, neurological, and gastrointestinal symptoms. Appears to be aging rapidly. Heavily medicated. Hitler at expected life expectancy with PD and CAD.	Catastrophic defeat of German forces at Stalingrad. Hitler refuses tactical retreats. Mental inflexibility. Allies invade Sicily, leading to collapse of Mussolini's regime.
June 1944	PD-related sleep disorder and violent outbursts prevent Hitler's awakening during early stages of D-Day. Mental rigidity slows assimilation of new information. Heavily medicated.	June 6, 1944, D-Day invasion at Normandy. Allies succeed in invasion, establish second front. Slow to release German reinforcements. The second front likely determines Germany's loss of World War II.
July 1944	Assassination attempt renders Hitler temporarily deaf, bleeding from ears, and splinters in legs. Heavily medicated.	Failed assassination by Col. Claus von Stauffenberg caused by Hitler's failure to follow advice of his generals in a timely way.
1945	Progression of chronic diseases. Hitler loses ability to sort through conflicting information and is physically limited. Increasingly mentally rigid, paranoid, reclusive, and angry.	Despite overwhelming odds and loss of military forces, Germany continues hopeless war. Orders scorched earth policy.
April 30, 1945	Hitler commits suicide in the Führerbunker.	Berlin overrun by Soviet Red Army. Germany sues for peace.

FOREWORD

To many of us, Adolf Hitler is a larger-than-life, monstrously malign madman, akin to a wickedly evil villain in a far-from-funny comic book. In our minds, he is a caricature, more myth than reality. We tend to forget that Adolf Hitler was a real person, just like the rest of us, with the baggage—both emotional and physical—that we all, to varying degrees, bring into and acquire during our journey through this world. Who we are and what we become are the consequences of multiple factors. Some traits, genetically gifted to us by our parents or imprinted upon us by the environment into which we are born and raised, we cannot control. Others are of our own making.

In this book, these factors are dissected under the steady hand of an individual uniquely equipped and qualified to wield the investigative scalpel. Dr. Tom Hutton is an internationally known and respected clinical neurologist whose career focused on the diagnosis and treatment of movement disorders, such as Parkinson's disease. What sets him apart from the rest of us with similar neurological training is his additional background in behavioral neurology, which included time spent training under the world-renowned neuropsychologist and father of modern neuropsychological assessment, Dr. Alexander Luria. Thus, Adolf Hitler, with his complex combination of physical, neurological, and emotional disorders and derangements, is a perfect case study for Dr. Hutton's professional eye.

Dr. Hutton can describe and explain calmly and precisely, in readily understandable and easily digestible wording, the factors that combined to form—or more accurately, deform—Hitler's personality and guide his actions. The Hutton searchlight illuminating childhood factors and events experienced by a young Adolf Hitler land not only on Hitler's parents, his home environment, and his school experiences but even extends to his psychiatrically afflicted, schizophrenic aunt. He also skillfully guides us through Hitler's teenage and young adult years, tracing the scars left by his experiences in Vienna and subsequently during World War I. However, it is in discussing and explaining Hitler's mounting medical issues and ailments, real and imagined, that Dr. Hutton provides an especially fascinating, cogent, and incisive analysis of the multiple medical and neurological disease processes that likely progressively impacted Hitler's ability to function and lead the German war effort and the German state itself, especially during the later stages of World War II. Of these, the description of the effects of his inexorably and relentlessly progressive Parkinson's disease is distinctly riveting.

Parkinson's disease (along with other forms of parkinsonism) often is a rare neurological disorder, and since it affects only about one in one thousand individuals in the general population, that is not an inaccurate assessment. However, it also is not the full picture. Parkinson's disease is an age-related disorder—if attention is focused on individuals aged sixty or above, the percentage of individuals affected by Parkinson's disease changes dramatically, moving from one in one thousand in the general population to one of every one hundred individuals in that age group. It so happens that most political leaders also fit into this age group, and, in fact, an impressive array of politicians has been diagnosed with Parkinson's disease (although, it must be noted, not necessarily during the time they were in office). Francisco Franco, Mao Zedong, Deng Xiaoping, George H. W. Bush, Eugene McCarthy, Pierre Trudeau, Yasser Arafat, George Wallace, Janet Reno, Pope John Paul II, Rev. Jesse Jackson, and, of course, Adolf Hitler all were diagnosed with Parkinson's disease or another form of parkinsonism.

The question of Adolf Hitler's Parkinson's disease has fascinated neurologists for many years. The physical manifestations of the disorder, especially the tremor but also other changes in motor function—such as reduced facial expression, impaired speech volume and articulation, stooped posture, reduced arm swing when walking, flexed posture of the arm, and slowed shuffling gait—have been evident in film clips and noted in reports penned by others before Dr. Hutton. But the issue of how some of the so-called nonmotor features of Parkinson's disease might have affected the way Hitler thought and acted as the war—and his disorder—progressed has received relatively little attention and provides fertile ground for the analysis presented by Dr. Hutton.

One nonmotor feature of Parkinson's disease, cognitive and behavioral dysfunction, is particularly important when considering the potential impact of Parkinson's disease on Adolf Hitler and, in turn, the world and is treated in impressive detail by Dr. Hutton in this book. His characterization of the effects that Parkinson's disease-induced cognitive and behavioral dysfunction may have had on Hitler's behavior and decision-making, notably during the waning stages of the war, is absolutely fascinating and instructive. While it is quite easy to observe and understand the effect that a catastrophic precipitous or acute medical process, such as the stroke suffered by Franklin Delano Roosevelt, may have on world events, it is easy to overlook and not fully consider the effect that gradually progressive medical disorders, especially chronic neurodegenerative diseases that evolve through years, may have on our national leaders and, consequently, on world events.

Another chronic medical problem experienced by Adolf Hitler, and described in some detail by Dr. Hutton, was bowel dysfunction, possibly representing irritable bowel syndrome. Although of interest, it is worth noting that bowel dysfunction in the form of constipation is one of the most frequent nonmotor features of Parkinson's disease and has been known to develop as much as two decades before the classic motor features of Parkinson's disease make their appearance. Individuals with chronic constipation have an increased risk of developing Parkinson's disease. There also is a growing literature documenting alterations of the bacterial flora of the intestinal tract (called the gut microbiome) with associated inflammation within the intestine in persons with Parkinson's disease, and it has been suggested that this may be where the pathology of Parkinson's disease first appears, before spreading to the brain. Hitler's gastrointestinal difficulties certainly entailed more than simple constipation, prompting the suggestion of irritable bowel syndrome, but it is very interesting to note that recently it has been reported that individuals with irritable bowel syndrome also are at increased risk of developing Parkinson's disease. Thus, these two chronic medical problems experienced by Adolf Hitler may conceivably have been related.

Dr. Hutton also describes in some detail the potential effects of the many medications with which Hitler's personal physician, Dr. Morell, plied him. It is of interest that the use of Mutaflor, one of the remedies provided by Dr. Morell for treatment of Hitler's gastrointestinal dysfunction and described by Dr. Hutton as "an emulsion of a particular strain of bacteria taken from the feces of healthy Bulgarian peasants," actually might be considered a primitive form of or attempt at what is now called fecal microbiome transplantation, which recently has been utilized as an experimental treatment for both irritable bowel syndrome and Parkinson's disease. Thus, in this regard Dr. Morell may prove to have been, although unwittingly, ahead of his time.

Realizing how Hitler's medical and neurological derangements may have altered the course of world history is both compelling and sobering. Bearing in mind the list of other politicians, detailed above, who also were diagnosed with Parkinson's disease or other forms of parkinsonism, one wonders what effect, if any, their neurological disorder may have had on their actions. Furthermore, given that this commentary is being published following a presidential election in the United States in which both candidates are well beyond seventy years of age and concerns about behavioral or cognitive impairment were suggested or implied regarding each candidate, consideration of the potential effect of chronic neurological and behavioral disorders on the function of political leaders may be more than just an interesting historical exercise.

RONALD F. PFEIFFER, MD
PROFESSOR, OHSU PARKINSON'S CENTER
DEPARTMENT OF NEUROLOGY
OREGON HEALTH AND SCIENCE CENTER

PREFACE

Describing the sizeable impact of Adolf Hitler's poor health and the desperate circumstances that existed in Germany following World War I represents the guiding light for writing this book. Much of the important information about *der Führer* currently resides in turgid historical tomes or psychologically related articles that prove confusing and off-putting for many readers. Nevertheless, the impact that Hitler's physical and mental health had on his conduct, especially during the latter phases of World War II, has relevance for a popular audience.

Even today, charismatic leaders from around the world increasingly undermine liberal democracies with their autocratic rule, ethnocentric views, xenophobia, hate-mongering, and stark cries of ultranationalism. Critically viewing the factors that contributed to the making of Adolf Hitler still has great currency today and provides further understanding of the enigmatic dictator.

Admittedly, researching Hitler's health for two decades has proved both enlightening and strangely taxing. Like a magnet with reversing polarity, I would initially feel a strong attraction to the fascinating enigma of the larger-than-life Adolf Hitler, only then to be repelled by his horrendous cruelty and prejudice—factors that unsettled more than a few nights' sleep. I came to wonder how such a physically unimposing man with such a limited education and unremarkable background could manage to spur a conflict-weary Germany to wage a war of annihilation, attempt to conquer most of Europe, and nearly put an end to the Western democracies. Like trade winds for ancient mariners, Hitler's failing health and historical influences steered his lifelong goals toward the rocky shoals of a galling and inevitable defeat.

I want to be upfront early on in this book that while Hitler's medical ailments in the last years of his life impeded his military and administrative performance, his neurological, cardiac, and gastrointestinal maladies did not cause his treachery. His traumatic upbringing and psychological pathologies had been laid down many years before his major medical disorders appeared. Hence, Hitler remains in this author's eyes fully culpable for the horrors he unleashed upon the world. How this formulation works out will be carefully detailed later in this work.

Hitler's political rise to chancellor proves fascinating, but even more so was his descent from the heights of power that coincided with his failing health. We are left to wonder: How had Hitler's grand plan for a "Greater Germany" gone so very wrong? Seeking to understand Germany's catastrophic strategic errors in World War II that relate to Hitler's deteriorating health status became the major focus of this book. Inevitably during a war, the emphasis lands on the leader of the country, especially when the leader happens to be a dictator.

Several principal questions cry out for answers: Why did Hitler launch the invasion of the Soviet Union in 1941 rather than await a full buildup of standard military munitions and the much-heralded "wonder weapons"? Why, as the tide of war inexorably turned against Germany, did Hitler increasingly frustrate the performance of his capable General Staff? Finally, why in the latter stages of the war had Hitler reacted so slowly to military reversals and to unleashing counterattacks?

From largely medical and behavioral perspectives these questions will be addressed throughout this volume. Scrutinizing Hitler from the viewpoint of his medical history provides insights into the man and his actions (or inactions). In medicine, taking a medical history from a patient is more than merely jotting down the History of the Present Illness (HPI) with symptom onset and rate of progression. It also includes a description of the patient's Past Medical Health (PMH) indicating illnesses that may relate to the current complaint or have influenced the patient's life in other ways. An understanding of Hitler's early health concerns, even those as minor as Hitler's happened to be, along with comprehending his unusual personality development, offers an intriguing backdrop for his adult decision-making and actions.

The taking of a medical history is a creative and exploratory exercise that provides suggestive material and is much like the task of a detective who hunts for clues in solving a crime. The significance of the clue may at first appear trivial and unimportant, only later to be valued by the sleuthhound for how it informs the final solution to the crime or medical diagnosis.

I am reminded of how my mentor A. R. Luria at the University of Moscow once responded during my fellowship on the US-USSR Health Exchange Program to my question as to what constituted good preparation for becoming a neuropsychologist. Surprisingly, the great Soviet Academician advised reading as many mysteries as possible, as he stated the sleuthing process for both neuropsychology and neurology was identical to that for detective work.

A medical history also includes a Family Health History (FHH). This aspect of a patient's medical history describes whether illnesses in family members had been contagious or inheritable. The many premature deaths in Hitler's family also aid our understanding of Hitler's overwrought health concerns and offer insights into his premonitions of an early death. The presence of tuberculosis in the Hitler family and Adolf's complaints of pulmonary disease require careful consideration. Adolf's fears also included whether he might have inherited "the Jewish disease" (syphilis) from his father. This concern resulted from the incorrect genetic beliefs of the time regarding syphilis transmission. How these fears affected his performance as the leader of Nazi Germany will play out in subsequent chapters.

Another aspect of a thorough medical history includes the patient's Social History (SH). Understanding the nature of personal relationships, economic circumstances, educational background, cultural influences, and the impact of alcohol, tobacco, or drug usage often provides useful diagnostic information. Like Hitler's family history, the social history of Hitler and the existing culture of the time yields valuable clues related to these major questions. Likewise, his use of excessive medications prescribed by his personal physician, Theodor Morell, and their potential harm will be discussed.

This structured approach to Hitler's medical circumstances guided me through my virtual medical evaluation of Adolf Hitler. This approach is how physicians think. It is how this author thinks. To avoid any confusion resulting from such medical terminology, additional terms more readily accessible to a nonmedical audience will also be used.

To comprehend Hitler's surprising attractiveness to the German people requires an understanding of the desperate times in which he lived. Tumultuous cultural disturbances in the early part of the twentieth century predicated Hitler's rise to power. The early twentieth century was a time of turmoil. Christianity, long a mainstay of European culture and values, was giving way to science and pseudoscience, old empires crumbled and new ones formed, and the worldwide Great Depression sent national economies reeling into free fall. The punitive conditions of the Treaty of Versailles that ended World War I placed enormous costs and burdens upon the German people. Germany suffered a collective despair, loss of autonomy, and national sense of injury. This simmering stew of unresolved grievances proved ripe for revolution and for the acceptance of a demagogue.

It was precisely at this fulcrum of history that Adolf Hitler began to trumpet his simplistic, populist catchphrases that promised the German people relief from the chaos of warring ideologies and their desperate struggles. Such political platitudes and scapegoating of Jews and other so-called undesirables along with a clarion call for *Lebensraum* ("living space") for a reborn "Greater Germany" proved irresistible to large numbers of fraught and despairing German citizens.

With so much already written about Hitler, some might ask what another book adds to our understanding of *der Führer*. Despite the voluminous historical material that exists about Hitler, much less attention has been devoted to his physical and mental health and the impact that his health had upon World War II. Much of the material that exists is old and medically out of date, calling for a fresher look at these aspects of Adolf Hitler's life.

In addition, many researchers have held reservations about labeling Hitler as either physically or mentally ill. These reservations have persisted due to an abundance of caution, fearing that medical or psychiatric diagnoses would somehow exculpate him from blame for the horrors of World War II. The formulation presented in the current volume in no way removes Hitler's culpability but clearly documents that Hitler was medically ill.

During my search for a clearer understanding of Hitler, I came across a long-running controversy between academic historians and behavioral scientists/physicians regarding their different approaches. World War II historians deal with old documents, war plans, diaries, and government records, and as such, they prefer concrete evidence to interpret Hitler's actions. At the same time, academic historians are not as well versed in the study of patterns of behavior or behavioral determinants, nor are they able to estimate the impact of Hitler's poor physical health. They also fear that the medical and behavioral labeling of Hitler would mitigate his guilt and that of the German citizenry that supported him.

On the other hand, psychologists, psychiatrists, and psychoanalysts have sought to understand the psychological drive behind Hitler's actions. In Hitler's case, understanding his unusual personality and declining health has merit for better understanding the "why" behind his actions. Yet such behavioral findings are not considered as "hard" evidence. It appears as if there has been missed communication between the two groups. Clearly both have information to explain the enigma that made Hitler who he was.

Hitler's major illnesses will be described and shown to have limited his life expectancy. Knowledge of his life-shortening illnesses provides insight into the timelines for specific military and political misadventures. An appreciation as to how chronic Parkinson's disease affects cognition, planning, and mental flexibility also will be shown to have special relevance for interpreting Hitler's judgment and slowness to respond militarily during his final years.

A few prominent people render history by their daring and skillful actions. Some notable individuals, however, were neither ethical nor moral in their pursuits. Some vainglorious history makers showed themselves to be categorically venal. Such was the case with Adolf Hitler—the man who became the face of evil for the twentieth century.

History has reviled Hitler's inhumanity and genocide. Such criticisms extend to Hitler's cavalier manipulation of science, distortion of Darwinism, misunderstanding of genetics, naïve claims of genetic purity, and hostile views as to how a self-described Aryan nation should interact with other nations and ethnicities whom they perceived as *Untermenschen* (inferior people). Nevertheless, when his actions are placed within the painful morass that faced Germany in the early part of the twentieth century, those actions, and the misplaced adoration of many of the German people, become easier to comprehend.

Despite the Western Allies' overwhelming military and economic strength, it can be argued that a very different postwar world may have come about had Hitler's policymaking and warmaking not been impaired by his physical and mental health. This book is principally about those medical and psychological factors internal to Hitler that played key roles in diminishing the clarity of his thought processes and how those factors impacted illustrative battles in World War II.

World War II historians have always tried to understand Hitler's questionable decision-making. My training in how brain illnesses alter cognitive behavior provides insights into Hitler's actions and his surprising inactions. While the behavioral impacts of chronic Parkinson's disease have been described during the last twenty-five years, their consequences for Hitler have not been carefully explored. Likewise, the impacts of Hitler's chronic coronary artery disease and his many minor illnesses along with Hitler's hypochondriasis have not been well woven into the historical tapestry of World War II.

My background as a clinical and research neurologist lies in interpreting medical and scientific findings. I have tried to relate generally accepted historical truths. But I have also incorporated additional interpretation, where appropriate, as to how Hitler's physical and emotional health may have contributed to his poor decision-making and how these factors relate to selected historical events.

While I did not have the opportunity to personally take a medical history or perform a physical examination of Adolf Hitler, extensive medical records and newsreels exist that nicely externalize his neurological disease. In addition, reports by several of his closest advisors and Hitler's personal physician allow for a reasonably complete medical record that includes his heart, neurological, and

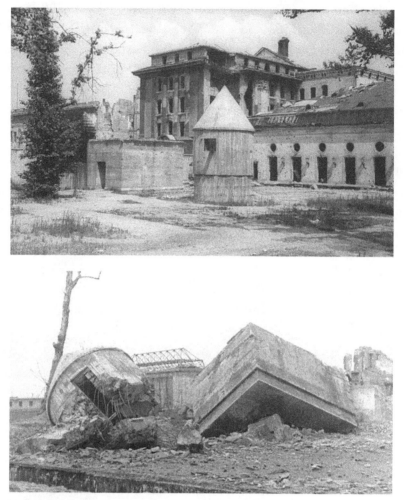

Top: The Führerbunker lay at the base of the Reich Chancellery. Hitler took up residence on January 16, 1945, and lived there until his death on April 30, 1945. (Bundesarchiv Bild 183-V04744). Bottom: Destroyed Führerbunker. The Soviets leveled the bunker and the site remained unmarked until 2006 when a small plaque marking the spot was added. (Bundesarchiv Bild 183-M1204-318 / Donath, Otto / CC-BY-SA 3.0)

gastrointestinal symptoms along with other minor illnesses. We also now have the results of his autopsy to mull, especially when trying to separate medical fact from Soviet political misinformation and propaganda.

In my earlier book, *Carrying the Black Bag: A Neurologist's Bedside Tales*, a chapter was devoted to the impact that Parkinson's disease had on Adolf Hitler's thought processes and the consequences that this medical entity had for the Battle of Normandy. Friends, colleagues, and my editor were intrigued and encouraged me to enlarge this approach into a full-length book to present a broader survey of the impact of Hitler's physical and mental health on World War II.

Hopefully this medical approach will provide further insight into the enigma that was Adolf Hitler and allow readers a more complete understanding of what drove the man to seek power and what health and historical factors ultimately brought him crashing down. If so, then writing this book will have proven a most worthwhile endeavor.

TOM HUTTON, MD, PHD
FREDERICKSBURG, TEXAS

ACKNOWLEDGMENTS

Many people are involved in publishing a book and justly deserve credit for their efforts. My sincere thanks go to those early readers of the manuscript including Janet Lindemann, La Nelle Etheridge, Tom Norris, and Madeline Douglass. Once again, I have turned to the very capable Maryglenn McCombs Warnock for publicity. She is an absolute pleasure with whom to work and continues to discover hidden gems within the domain of publicity.

I also express special thanks to my patient wife Trudy for her willingness to read drafts, retrieve photos and permissions, and create a helpful index. All through the process Trudy has provided encouragement for this challenging project. Knowing fully that an author should never, ever ask a spouse for such services, I again capitulated, fully realizing the immense value of her assistance.

Also, I wish to acknowledge the wonderful people working at Texas Tech University Press. After all, it was Joanna Conrad, the managing director, who first encouraged me to write this book. It then became the task of the acquisitions editor, Travis Snyder, to work through two to three years of daunting COVID-19 lockdowns and inconveniences. Travis never gave up on this project despite limited staff, working from home, having trouble locating homebound reviewers, incurring supply chain disruptions, and facing soaring publishing costs. The length of time for my book to be reviewed doubled and would have been even greater without Travis's steadfastness to see the process through. Finally, I thank John Brock for his experienced hand in marketing and his efforts in getting the book before the reading public and also Carly Kahl for copyediting. The professionalism of these and others at TTU Press made this a better book.

Many friends and supporters, too numerous to mention, have encouraged my writing efforts. Such valuable aid and emotional support are acknowledged and appreciated more than you will ever know.

As my book is released during the 100th anniversary of the founding of Texas Tech, it is appropriate that I thank the institution from which I graduated so many years ago. When I attended Tech, it was a small college that lay in the center of the small, gusty, dusty city of Lubbock. When this wannabe doctor first headed west to Lubbock to study pre-med, never would I have imagined how well Texas Tech would prepare me for my career in medicine or how this affordable and public state-supported college would grow into the outstanding educational institution that it has become. Years later when I returned to Texas Tech's medical school serving as Vice Chair of Medical and Surgical Neurology, I recognized the excellent medical center that Lubbock was developing that included the largest hospital between Dallas and Los Angeles. Much later during retirement, I again found myself associated with Tech through my volunteer efforts to develop its regional teaching site in Fredericksburg, Texas.

From its humble and unpretentious beginning, Texas Technological College has grown into a system that now includes Texas Tech University, an internationally known and respected institution of higher learning with enrollment of more than 40,000 students; Angelo State University; Midwestern State University; two health science centers; a law school; and a School of Veterinary Medicine. Furthermore, demonstration of its excellence stems from Tech achieving tier one research university status, a highly respected graduate school, and fifteen locations, among them Lubbock, Texas; Seville, Spain; and San José, Costa Rica. This current bustling public university, nevertheless, continues to produce determined, hardworking, independent-minded, and well-trained graduates that today carry the Tech banner far and wide. It is only fitting that I recognize the indelible impact that Texas Tech University has made upon my life.

Paul Whitfield Horn, the first president of Texas Tech, in a 1926 speech expressed his thoughts on Texas Tech that are just as true one hundred years hence as they were then:

> It is a magnificent country in which our college is located, it is a region of magnificent distances, of far-flung horizons, of deep canyons, of lofty far-arching skies. Everything that is done on these West Texas Plains ought to be on a big scale. It is a country that lends itself to bigness. It is a country that does not harmonize with things little or narrow or mean. Let us make the work of our college fit into the scope of our country. Let our thoughts be big thoughts. Let our thinking be in world-wide terms.

Congratulations, Texas Tech University, on your one hundredth birthday, and a big THANK YOU for giving me my start in higher education.

HITLER'S MALADIES

AND THEIR IMPACT ON WORLD WAR II

CHAPTER 1

THE EARLY YEARS

A Past Medical Health (PMH), as noted in the preface, begins with the patient's birth and proceeds to describe early development. Any records, if they even existed, of Klara Hitler's birth to Adolf have been lost to history. What is known is that she was in good health at the time of Adolf's birth. Anesthetics were not in common usage, so the process likely proved agonizing for Klara.

She was an experienced mother, having previously given birth to two children. Births in the 1880s usually occurred at home with the help of family or friends. Whether a midwife or a physician attended her in Braunau am Inn, Austria, for Adolf's birth is unknown but unlikely. It is reasonable to assume given her good health and prior unremarkable birth of two children that Adolf's birth also was unremarkable. The PMH for Adolf starts with what little is known about his birth and early development.

BIRTH AND BIRTHPLACE

As the sun descended toward the dark part of Saturday, April 20, 1889, a little-noted event occurred that ultimately impacted the entire world. For at that time Adolfus Hitler, as his name was listed on his birth certificate, was born at Salzburger Vorstadt 15 in Braunau am Inn. No one could have predicted that the angelic, blue-eyed infant would one day become the most hated man in history or that he would trigger the deaths of more than fifty million people.

For the first three years of his life, Adolf's family lived in Braunau am Inn. They resided in a modest guesthouse while Adolf's father worked as a minor Austrian customs official at the nearby Austria–Germany border. Years later, the guesthouse became a government facility, a bank, a technical school, and a library. In 1989, exactly 100 years following Hitler's birth, the mayor of Braunau am Inn placed a somber memorial stone at the previously unmarked site of Hitler's birth. Translated it reads, "For Peace, Freedom, and Democracy. Never Again Fascism. Millions of Dead Remind." The stone for the memorial carries with it a sad irony, as it was quarried at the former Mauthausen concentration camp that is located not far from Braunau am Inn.

In 1938, Martin Bormann (head of the Nazi Party Chancellery) purchased for the Nazi Party the building in which Adolf Hitler had been born. For a time during the Third Reich, the structure became a gathering place and a shrine for the Nazi cult. Following World War II, the building briefly housed Allied soldiers. Only in 2016 did the Austrian government schedule demolition of Hitler's birthplace to prevent it from ever becoming a rallying point for neo-Nazis or an unintended shrine to Adolf Hitler. Later developments suggested that rather than being torn down, it should be remodeled and no longer left recognizable as Hitler's birthplace. In 2020, Austria unveiled a new design for the location by turning it into a police station.

In the twenty-first century, Braunau am Inn contains some sixteen thousand people. It is surrounded by majestic green spaces, a river, and burbling streams. In 1890, around the time that Adolf Hitler was born, it was smaller and even more pristine than it is now and boasted a population of only 5,584. It is hard to envision the malevolence that Hitler would unleash on the world as occurring from such an unspoiled, bucolic environment.

HITLER'S PARENTS

At the time of his birth, Hitler's parents were a fifty-two-year-old alcoholic doctrinaire customs officer by the name of Alois Hitler and a twenty-nine-year-old poorly educated but loving Klara Hitler. Klara first came to Alois Hitler's home by working as his servant and then served as a nursemaid for Alois's second wife, Fanny, who suffered and eventually died from tuberculosis. Klara became Alois's mistress, became pregnant by him, and gave birth to Gustav in May 1885. Following Fanny's death in August 1884, Klara and Alois married in January 1885. It was Alois's third marriage.

Since Alois and Klara were second cousins, they had to petition the Catholic Church for special dispensation to marry. The Church sensibly held the view that close relatives should not marry due to the increased risk of congenital malformations in their offspring. It would seem logical that Klara's obvious pregnancy and overt need for financial support should have compelled the Church to sanction their marriage, seeing it as the lesser of two evils. Nevertheless, Alois in his petition

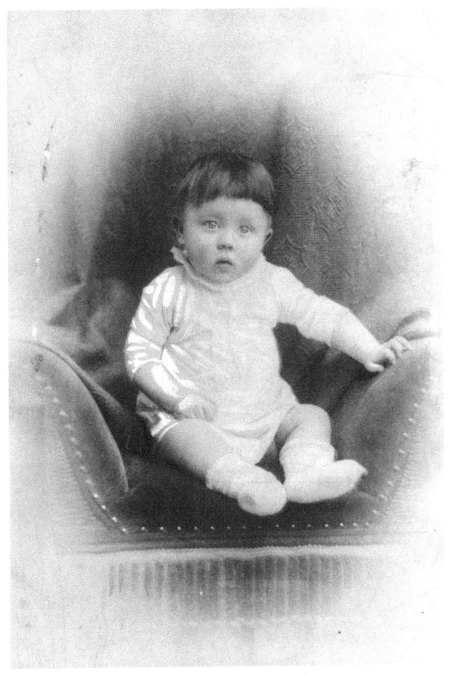

Adolf Hitler as an infant. (Bundesarchiv Bild 183-1989-0322-506)

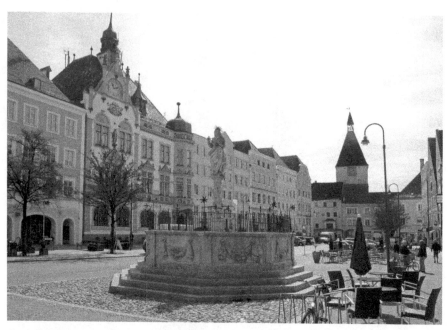

Central square in Braunau am Inn, the Austrian city where Adolf Hitler was born. (Stadtamt Braunau am Inn, CC BY-SA 3.0)

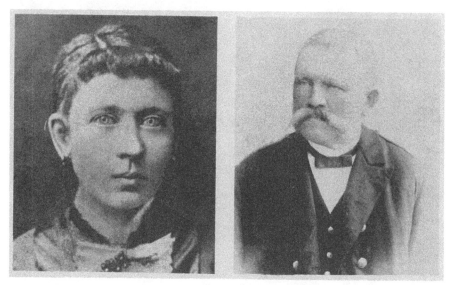

Klara Hitler on the left—his mother, whom Adolf loved—and the stern father, Alois Hitler, on the right, whom Adolf hated. (Kara Hitler LC-USZ62-44197, Lot 4890; Alois Hitler, LC-USZ62-44196)

conveniently failed to even mention Klara's pregnancy and instead implored the Church to grant what he saw as his greatest need, a mother for his children. His request was all about Alois's needs. It suggests Alois's egocentricity, a characteristic that would later become equally obvious in his son, Adolf. The Catholic Church eventually relented on its proscription against related people marrying and approved Alois and Klara's application for marriage.

PARENTAL AND CHILD RELATIONSHIPS

Hitler revealed his feelings for his parents in his political screed, *Mein Kampf*, where he wrote, "I honored my Father, but I loved my Mother." Young Adolf respected but feared his father, an authoritarian, demanding, and abusive parent. But at the same time, he deeply loved his mother. His parents were in some ways opposites.

Alice Miller, a psychoanalyst and author, provides in her 1980 book, *For Your Own Good*, a strong argument for Adolf having been physically and emotionally abused by his father. She describes the potential damage resulting from child abuse ("poisonous pedagogy" was the phrase she used) and examined Adolf Hitler as an example of such a bad outcome. It was her belief that human destructiveness is a reactive, not an innate, phenomenon. Certainly not all children who have endured corporal punishment or even more pronounced child abuse have suffered such severe psychological impacts or performed such horrendous deeds as did Hitler.

Miller drew heavily on biographical and historical material from John Toland (*Adolf Hitler*, Vol. 1, 1976) and Joachim Fest (*Hitler*, 1974). She described how Hitler's father frequently whipped and humiliated Adolf, creating deep psychological scars in the boy that she claimed later fueled his penchant for aggression and violence. She proposes that by humiliating young Adolf, Alois created a smoldering, pent-up rage in his son that one day he would vent upon the world.

The wife of Hitler's Harvard-educated foreign press secretary, Ernst "Putzi" Hanfstaengl, shared with Toland the "Toga Boy" story. This tantalizing anecdote, according to Miller, encapsulates the humiliation young Adolf suffered from his overbearing and authoritarian father. As the story goes, because of his many frustrations and arguments with his father, young Adolf determined to run away from home. Alois learned of his son's plans to sneak off and thwarted them by locking Adolf in an upstairs room that had bars across its windows. The rebellious, slender Adolf tried to escape by wriggling between the bars in the window. He found the opening between the bars barely too small to squirm through, so Adolf backed off, removed his clothing, and reattempted his escape. It was during the act of trying

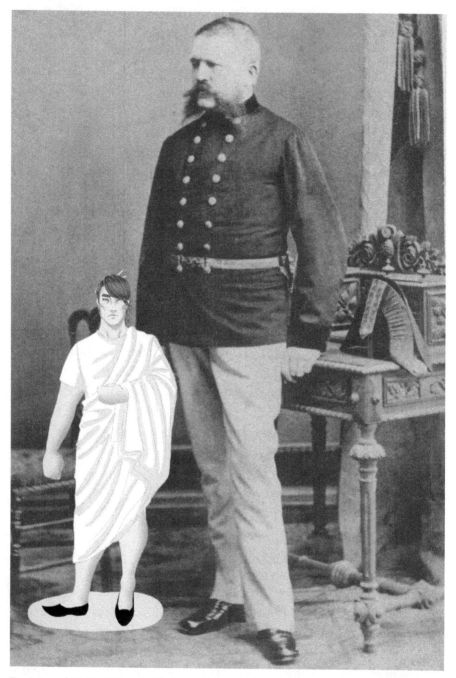

Depiction of Adolf as "Toga Boy," who was humiliated by his father, Alois. (Alois Hitler, Alamy stock photo)

to squirm naked between the bars that Adolf heard his father's heavy bootsteps ominously ascending the narrow wooden stairway. Adolf quickly aborted his attempted flight, jumped to the floor, and hastily covered his nakedness with an available tablecloth.

On entering the room and seeing his son with a tablecloth draped around him toga-style, Alois threw back his head and guffawed at his son's ridiculous appearance. Rather than whipping the boy, he determined to humiliate him. Alois called for Klara, and in front of his wife further ridiculed the silly toga-like appearance of their son. Alois demanded Klara take a long look at "Toga Boy."

No doubt Alois also noticed Adolf's discarded clothes that had been strewn hastily about the floor. He may have even revealed Adolf's nudity to his mother. If so, to the excessively modest Adolf (described later when the adult Hitler refused to disrobe even for his personal doctor), such exposure would have been utterly mortifying. His father's protracted belittling of Adolf lasted for days, and this prolonged ridicule came from the very man whose love Adolf most craved. This parental belittling had a crushing effect on the young artistic boy's spirit.

Alice Miller held that such humiliation as revealed in the Toga Boy story proved more destructive for Adolf than would have the switch. Years later, Adolf confided that it took him a very long time to recover from this episode of ridicule, humiliation, and embarrassment.

Helm Stierlin, in his 1976 book, *Adolf Hitler: A Family Perspective*, provides further evidence of Adolf's rebelliousness. While in Realschule (roughly the equivalent of high school), he was known to mock his teachers and perform silly, attention-seeking pranks. On one occasion he showed extreme disregard for the school's authority by using his report card in lieu of toilet paper to wipe himself. Such was the low regard young Adolf had for school, its rules, and his teachers.

Adolf harbored a deep hatred of his father; nevertheless, he treated Alois Sr. with the great respect the older man demanded. Adolf Hitler even referred to his father quite formally in *Mein Kampf* as *Herr Vater*. Young Adolf lived with Alois's reproaches and knew that despite anything he might do to gain that parent's love, nothing would prevent his father's nearly daily thrashings, frequent humiliation, and seemingly loveless relationship.

Alois had no great attachment to, nor derived satisfaction from, any of his children apart from his youngest child, Paula. Adolf's youthful disregard for authority regularly raised the ire of his doctrinaire, rule-following father. Alois was alarmed and outraged by his rebellious and disobedient sons, Adolf and Alois Jr., Adolf's older half-brother. Alois Sr. practiced the severe child-rearing methods of the day that were common in Austria and Germany—that is, "spare the rod and spoil the child"—with Alois Jr. receiving most of the physical punishment. Considerable controversy exists as to whether Adolf received any greater physical discipline than did other German or Austrian children at the time.

Alice Miller, drawing heavily from John Toland, posits that Adolf did receive severe beatings by his outraged, out-of-control father. She makes the point that a beaten child who then is forced to stifle his feelings will later find a way to release these suppressed emotions.

Alois Jr., Adolf's half-brother, and Adolf's younger sister, Paula, provided corroboration of Adolf's mistreatment by his father. After World War II, both siblings shared their reminiscences of mistreatment and whippings of Adolf, when hostility toward Hitler and Germany was prevalent and could have brought about exaggeration of their accounts. According to Toland, Alois Jr. claimed that Alois Sr. beat Adolf unmercifully with a hippopotamus whip. The adult Adolf Hitler also shared stories with his secretaries of his mistreatment by his father; however, Hitler is known to have told fanciful stories to them on other topics.

In any event, Miller believed that the father's demeaning treatment and humiliation of Adolf along with stifling the boy's feelings may have inculcated his intense lifelong, insatiable hatred that in later years he would spew out upon the world. Adolf's mother proved helpless to prevent such child abuse, as Alois Sr. would, if interfered with, turn his rage on Klara and beat her as well. Klara's lack of emotional support during these beatings further added to the throttling of Adolf's ability to work through his psychological turmoil.

Alois Hitler Sr. exhibited an uncompromising stubbornness in his child-rearing practices that would later become a personality characteristic in his son, Adolf. Alois Sr. was intransigent and could not be guided toward tolerance by family, friends, or others. Moreover, his stubbornness was accompanied by both intimidating anger and violent outbursts.

Numerous psychological studies exist today that show how such ongoing harsh and abusive treatment of children can create disastrous results in a child's developing personality. These features include learning problems, difficulty relating to peers, oppositional defiant behaviors, conduct disorder, aggression, depression, and anxiety, among others. To a degree, Adolf Hitler as a youth demonstrated these personality characteristics.

These abuses by Alois Sr. were often prompted by Adolf's goal of becoming an artist rather than a civil servant like his father, according to Brigitte Hamann in her 1999 book *Hitler's Vienna: A Dictator's Apprenticeship*. The author also shared Alois Sr.'s frustration with Adolf's failure to sustain hard work. Adolf's vocational interests further mystified his practical-minded father. After years of struggle Alois Sr. eventually relented and enrolled Adolf in a technical drawing school, although likely hoping that Adolf would become a technical artist and not a fine artist. Adolf's stubbornness, patterned after his father's behavior, may also have reminded Alois of his own personal shortcomings.

Scapegoating was another prominent defense mechanism frequently employed by Alois Sr., one that young Adolf regularly witnessed and adopted. Adolf learned this technique well, often blaming his siblings or playmates for breakage of items, accidents, or incidents that Adolf had in fact caused. Of possible significance is that later scapegoating became evident in Adolf's political life when he blamed Jews, homosexuals, the intelligentsia, and communists for various misdeeds, some of which Hitler and his Nazi Party members had clandestinely fomented. Later in life Hitler was known to sack senior officers for military failures rather than accept blame for his own strategic and tactical mistakes.

ADOLF'S PLAYMATES AND SIBLINGS

According to Toland, Adolf's bossiness and penchant for giving impassioned speeches to his playmates and family foreshadowed his later behavior as an adult. Also, his awkward social interaction with his playfellows identifies why Adolf, for the most part, had difficulty establishing meaningful relationships as a youth, an experience that also played out later in his life.

According to Fritz Redlich, a psychiatrist who wrote the 1999 book *Diagnosis of a Destructive Prophet*, between the ages of five and eight Adolf referred to himself as a "little gang leader." The young Adolf enjoyed playing war games, focusing particularly on the Boer War in Africa or what he referred to as his "Indian and Trapper" game. Even as a boy, war in various forms held a certain fascination for Adolf. Certainly, playing war games or "cowboys and Indians" games was not unusual at the time among children, but it does provide evidence of an early attraction toward conflict in young Adolf.

Dietrich Güstrow (a pen name) gave us "The Billy Goat Story" as described in Hans-Joachim Neumann and Henrik Eberle's 2013 book *Was Hitler Ill?* Güstrow said that he had heard the story from Eugen Wasner, a former childhood friend of Hitler and a German soldier in World War II. While on the Eastern Front, Wasner enjoyed entertaining his fellow soldiers with tales about their *Führer* when he was but an impudent boy.

Among those stories was the description of when a young Adolf and friends in 1895 or 1896 pried open the mouth of a billy goat and wedged a stick between its jaws. Adolf then proceeded to pee into the goat's mouth. The episode came to an unfortunate outcome for Adolf, as the startled goat responded by biting through the wedged stick and down on Adolf's penis. Adolf's shriek in response to his pain no doubt provided further entertainment for his playmates and later to Wasner's fellow soldiers.

While undoubtedly amused by such ribald tales, the well-disciplined German soldiers felt compelled to report Lance Corporal Wasner's intemperate and disrespectful stories to their superiors. This information led to Wasner's arrest and to his standing trial. In 1943, while under interrogation, Wasner failed to recant the episodes that he had previously disclosed to his fellow soldiers.

According to Güstrow, who served as Wasner's attorney, the verdict read by the chairman of the tribunal was as follows: "In the name of the people: The accused Eugen Wasner has treacherously and in the worst of manners insulted and slandered Germany's *Führer* and Chancellor of the Reich. He has hereby and by other defeatist statements corrupted the military strength of the German people. He will therefore be punished with the death sentence. The trial is closed; the accused is to be taken into custody." Wasner was beheaded by guillotine in Berlin Plötzensee some forty-five years following Hitler's silly childhood prank with the billy goat.

Wasner's story demonstrates at least two major points. The first was Hitler's meanness to an animal, although this example seems to be the only documented incident of animal cruelty, and he was certainly later in life known to lavish love on his dogs and even showed concern for crustaceans. The second major point was the lengths to which the Third Reich would resort to prevent *der Führer* from being placed in an unfavorable light, including use of the guillotine for such petty offenses.

The story also adds questionable support for the notion that Adolf Hitler might have had mutilation of his genitals, although historians have largely discounted this claim. Most authors have rejected the speculation about Hitler's genital damage with its purported relationship to his anti-Semitism (more about this topic in chapter 9).

Returning to Adolf's immediate family history, four of his full siblings—Gustav, Ida, Otto, and Edmund—all died young, causing their mother, Klara, immeasurable grief. Adolf was the middle child among them. Gustav (born May 17, 1887; died December 18, 1887) and Ida (born September 1886; died January 2, 1888) were his older siblings. Otto (born June 17, 1892; died June 23, 1892) and Edmund (born March 24, 1894; died February 2, 1900) were his younger siblings.

All are believed to have died from diphtheria (or possibly measles in Edmund's case), a bacterial infection for which an effective vaccine was not invented until 1921 but did not go into widespread usage until the 1930s. Of Klara's children, only Adolf and his younger sister Paula survived to adulthood. Premature deaths of his four siblings psychologically impacted Adolf. These losses likely encouraged the notion that he somehow was special and had survived for a good reason. It may have also underscored his later belief that he, like most of his siblings and his mother, would not live into old age.

ADOLF'S LOVING RELATIONSHIP WITH HIS MOTHER AND AMBIVALENCE TOWARD HIS HALF-SIBLINGS

It is hard to fathom the depth of the tragedy for Klara from having four of her children die, and in a fairly short period of time. The extent of Klara's grief must have been profound. Paula was born when Adolf was seven years old. Her birth prompted Adolf's removal from the parental bedroom to make room for the younger Edmund and Paula.

Following the deaths of four of her children, Klara increasingly doted on her remaining child, Adolf. Prior to the birth of her youngest child, Paula, her mothering energies and desperate hopes for redemption for her emotionally and socially impoverished life had been focused entirely on her young son. It was in him that she held her fondest hopes for the justification of her life.

One can imagine her conscious or subconscious desperation in placing her expectations on her lone surviving son. Her spoiling of Adolf knew no bounds, as she would even condone Adolf's skipping school and failure to do his homework. Such constant fawning must have inculcated in Adolf a belief that he was somehow special and that he could choose not to abide by the rules that others in society must follow.

Further development of Hitler's egoism occurred over the years that allowed his feelings of childhood impunity to morph into his adult messianic belief that he, and only he, was destined to address Germany's political difficulties. How Hitler came to believe that he alone would be capable of delivering Germany from its harsh economic and political woes will be discussed further in the next chapter.

Adolf's relationship with his undistinguished half-siblings, Alois Jr. and Angela, was ambivalent, if not downright antagonistic. His relationship with his younger sister Paula also became strained when Adolf later lost his orphan's pension in a legal action to Paula. The pension had been a major source of his support as an adolescent in Vienna and had supplemented his mother's generosity. Following

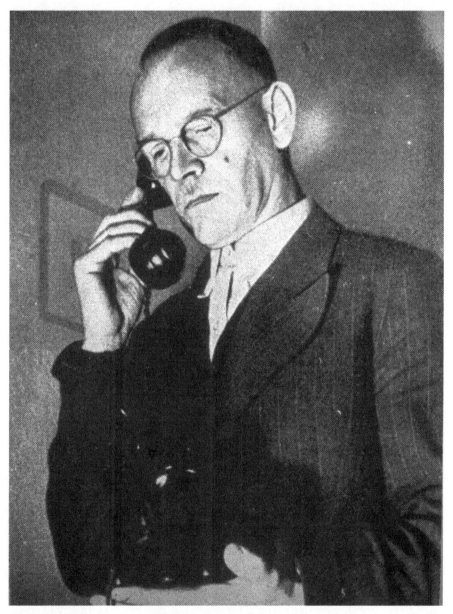

Alois Hitler Jr., Adolf's half-brother. (Alamy stock photo)

the loss of the pension, his income came from meager earnings from odd jobs, from painting postcards, and several loans from his maternal aunt, Johanna Pölzl.

Years later, Adolf Hitler rarely spoke of his half-siblings, and they played limited roles in his life. His half-brother Alois Jr. left home early and proved to be a colorful individual. He was charged and convicted of theft and imprisoned for five months

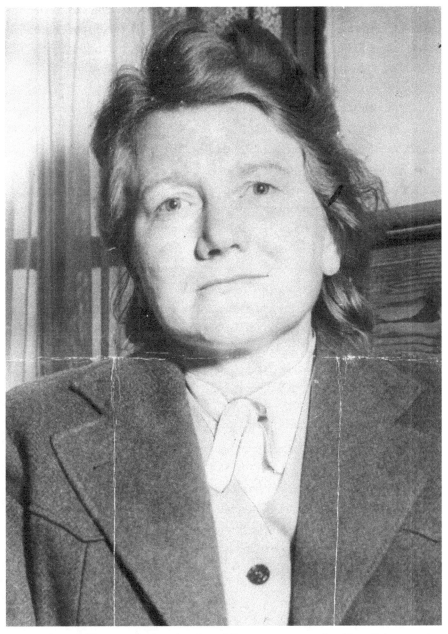

Paula Hitler, Adolf's younger sister, who after a falling-out over an orphans' benefit later reunited with Adolf and worked as his housekeeper. (Alamy stock photo)

in 1900 and then again for another eight months in 1902. In 1905 he obtained a job as a waiter in London. In 1909 Alois Jr. met an Irishwoman named Bridget Dowling. They married and settled in Liverpool. He attempted to make a living, but all his business dealings ended in failure. He then abandoned his Irish wife and son and returned to Germany to establish himself as a safety-razor salesman. He married again in Berlin and in 1924 was charged with bigamy. In 1934 he opened a restaurant in Berlin. According to Dr. Eduard Bloch, the Hitler family physician, Alois Jr. was never overly friendly with Adolf.

Older half-sister Angela for a time managed a restaurant for Jewish students at the University of Vienna. Angela, according to Walter Langer's 1972 wartime report *The Mind of Adolf Hitler*, once defended her Jewish residents from attack by Aryan rioters. In 1906 she married Leo Raubal, who was a junior tax inspector and who died in 1910. Adolf reestablished limited contact with Angela in 1919 and in 1928 she and her daughter Geli moved near Berchtesgaden where Angela became Hitler's housekeeper. She was later put in charge of the household. She and Adolf had a falling out over Eva Braun, and Angela left Berchtesgaden for Dresden. In 1936 Angela married an architect and professor in Dresden by the name of Martin Hammitzsch who later committed suicide following the defeat of Germany in World War II. Even after the war ended, Angela continued to speak highly of Adolf and maintained that neither she nor Adolf had known anything about the Holocaust.

Paula, Adolf's younger sister, did not marry. In 1930 she changed her name at Adolf's urging from Hitler to Wolf to be less conspicuous in public. She also began describing herself as "Mrs." to be even more incognito. These masquerades came about following Paula's having lost her job at a Viennese insurance agency in 1930 after her bosses learned the identity of her controversial brother. She worked as a secretary at a hospital during World War II. Paula is the only one of Adolf's siblings who in later years had more than a passing interaction with Adolf.

"He was still my brother, no matter what happened," Paula Hitler was quoted as saying. Uncannily she also said in an interview late in her life, "I must honestly confess that I would have preferred it if he had followed his original ambition and become an architect. . . . It would have saved the world a lot of worries." In this statement Paula Hitler poignantly speaks for a war-ravaged world and perhaps voices the understatement of the century.

CHAPTER 2

ADOLF'S ADOLESCENT BEHAVIOR

D uring Adolf Hitler's adolescence, significant health and behavioral developments occurred that would impact his character for a lifetime. His Family
Medical History (FMH), an outline of the medical illnesses occurring
within the family, may also have spurred his development of hypochondriasis.

UNUSUAL ADOLESCENT BEHAVIOR
In psychiatry the phrase "the child is father of the man" is commonly used to vividly describe childhood behaviors and experiences that impact the development
of the adult personhood. The catchy phrase, while co-opted by behaviorists, was
first used by William Wordsworth, the British Romanticist poet, in 1807 in a poem
entitled, "My Heart Leaps Up," also known as "The Rainbow."

Even early in his childhood, Adolf suffered anxiety, eating problems, temper
tantrums, and learning difficulties, all of which reflected upon his developing
personality. Adolf's eating and digestive problems, as it turned out, predicted a
lifetime of unpleasant gastrointestinal symptoms.

Adolf had a behaviorly troubled youth, and his youth spawned an even more
troubled adulthood. Robert G. L. Waite in his 1977 book *The Psychopathic God
Adolf Hitler* argues that Adolf must have grown up in a home charged with tension.
As psychoanalysts have previously noted, no person manifesting Adolf Hitler's
personality traits could possibly have been raised in the idyllic environment Hitler
liked to later paint for himself. Waite suggests that the constant threat of Alois's
temper played a major role in creating this friction. His father's temper combined
with Klara's struggle to control her emotions of guilt and disappointment and

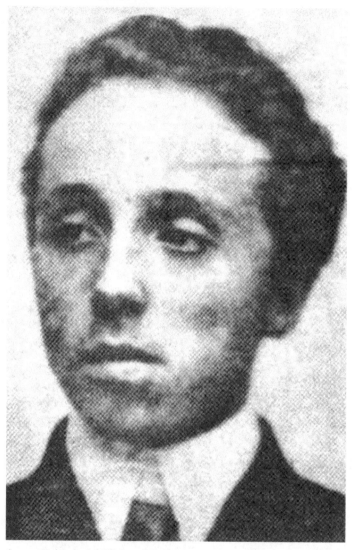

August Kubizek, Adolf's best friend growing up, who traveled to Vienna with him. (Alamy stock photo)

having to deal with her violent, largely uncommunicative husband further added to the family tension. Together these stressors created a strained childhood home that is believed to have triggered Adolf's troubled personality.

Adolf's scapegoating of his playmates and his frequent temper tantrums resulted in his largely becoming a loner. Most children simply could not tolerate his tantrums and were unwilling to submit to his bossiness. When Adolf was somewhat older an exception occurred in the person of August Kubizek.

August Kubizek, author of *The Young Hitler I Knew* (2011), was one of the very few friends during Adolf's late teenage years in Linz and later in Vienna. Kubizek described the extensive orations that young Adolf would deliver. These speeches usually occurred when the two teenagers were out walking. These verbal tirades could take the form of lectures on historical or political topics or could turn angry due to some trivial matters, such as young Hitler not getting his way. Adolf's unpredictable anger reminded his boyhood friend of an erupting volcano.

Nevertheless, Kubizek found Hitler's style of oratory nothing short of mesmerizing, deeming his delivery of a speech far superior to the words that Hitler uttered. This oratorical skill later became apparent in Hitler's political speeches, when the German people responded fervently to his orations but felt far less impressed when reading his words in the newspaper.

When Adolf determined to leave Linz for the big city of Vienna, he cajoled his friend August to go along with him so that Adolf could study at the Academy of Fine Arts while Kubizek studied at the Conservatory. On one occasion while in Vienna, Kubizek introduced Adolf to a girl from Silesia who had sought Kubizek's help in interpreting a difficult musical score. Adolf, who had recently been dropped by a girl he had liked, erupted in an emotional tirade, claiming the girl from Silesia must be infatuated with him. He continued his tirade by shouting that she should not have been studying at the Conservatory in any event since she was a girl. Hitler's misogyny that day was on full display. According to Kubizek:

> I had a job to convince him that the girl was not suffering from pangs of love, but from examination pains. The result was a detailed speech about the senselessness of women studying. Like blows the words fell on me, as though I were the cloth manufacturer or the brewer who had sent his daughter to the Conservatory. Adolf got himself more and more involved in a general criticism of social conditions. I cowered silently on the piano stool while he enraged, strode the three steps along and the three steps back and hurled his indignation in the bitterest terms, first against the door, and then against the piano.... He would fly into a temper at the slightest thing.

Even as a teenager Adolf had learned to direct Kubizek's emotions and had played on them effectively. This early talent in Hitler illustrates how later his political oratory held such great sway for desperate and war-weary Germans. In addition, Hitler was able to later assess and express the frustrations, fears, anxieties, hopes, and desires of the despondent German people. While Kubizek initially believed Adolf's speeches to be an act, as if Adolf were on stage, he later came to understand that Adolf was deadly earnest in his expressed beliefs. During these oratorical frenzies Adolf required Kubizek's unbridled adoration and later expected the same reaction from his German audiences.

While young Kubizek tolerated Hitler's domineering attitude surprisingly well, many others at the time found his behavior obnoxious. A tendency to tirades is, after all, not a particularly attractive feature in a teenage chum and explains, at least in part, why young Adolf had so few friends while growing up.

The young Adolf also showed early evidence of grandiosity. Despite struggling in school and while still living in Linz, the young Adolf determined to redesign and rebuild his hometown. Kubizek devoted a whole chapter in his book to Adolf's elaborate plans for his hometown of Linz: "The first time I went to visit him at home, his room was littered with sketches, drawings, blueprints. Here was the 'new theatre,' there the mountain hotel on the Lichtenberg—it was like an architect's office."

Adolf's facility with sketching and drawing architectural plans clearly impressed young Kubizek. Nevertheless, in the face of failing subjects in school, such impracticality as redesigning his hometown shows evidence not only of his aptitude for drawing architectural plans but also his early onset of vaingloriousness.

DEATH OF ADOLF'S FATHER

In 1903, when Adolf was in his early teens, his father, Alois, died from a presumed pulmonary hemorrhage. Knowing his father died such a violent death may have increased Adolf's concern about his own lung disease. The suddenness of his father's gory death may also have increased Adolf's fear of his own violent death.

Adolf's uncompromising and authoritarian father had often resorted to violence in an attempt both to achieve his work-related goals and to force his opinions on young Adolf. Some behavioral scientists hold that such a forceful parental attitude became a construct for an authoritarian political party and for a government that was quick to resort to violence to achieve its goals. The technique of using fear, intimidation, and violence that had been a parental tactic within the immediate Hitler family may have later become a model for Adolf Hitler's implementation of his fiercely held political goals.

A second factor that may have influenced Adolf's acceptance of violence will be dealt with in a later chapter on World War I when Adolf witnessed extensive human carnage. He saw many blood-soaked battlefields as he ran messages between headquarters and the German trenches. Such a horrific experience as trench warfare may also have inured Adolf to brutality in his later pursuit of Germany's national ambitions.

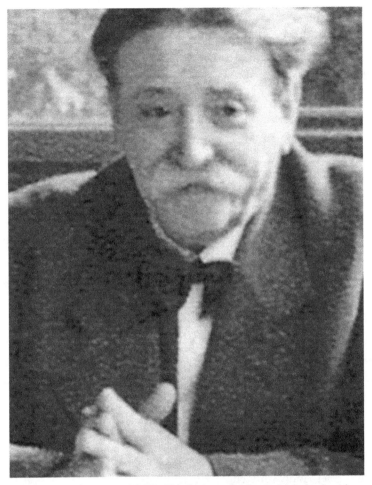

Dr. Eduard Bloch, whom Adolf held in high esteem despite his being Jewish and who provided valuable historical insights into Adolf's upbringing and the Hitler family. (Alamy stock photo)

IMPACT OF ADOLF'S MOTHER

As noted earlier, in contrast to his negative feelings toward his father, Adolf adored his mother, who basically spoiled him. Klara fawned on young Adolf, in part it is believed to counterbalance his father's punitive and demeaning conduct.

Klara was emotionally warm and socially adept. She made those around her feel comfortable and encouraged. Klara acted in a docile manner toward her husband and was thoroughly dominated by him.

Klara impressed Dr. Eduard Bloch, their family physician, as both a good mother and a tidy housekeeper. He wrote a two-part story titled "My Patient,

Hitler" that originally appeared in the March 15 and March 22, 1941, issues of *Collier's* magazine in which he detailed his relationship to the Hitler family and especially to young Adolf. Surprisingly, he found the young Adolf largely unremarkable and to be a polite and obedient boy. While appearing frail, the boy proved generally healthy, with only the usual colds, flu, and sore throats. Bloch acknowledged the father's attempt to control Adolf's future and to push him toward a stable government career. In response, Adolf became oppositional to his father's controlling manner, provoking many arguments in which Klara tried, but largely failed, to play the peacemaker.

Klara Hitler doted on young Adolf and supported his longing to become a visual artist. She, in contrast to her husband, complimented Adolf on his drawings and encouraged his artistic efforts. Following the death of Alois Sr., Klara sold the family farm and moved to the outskirts of Linz. There she bought a house and managed to raise the family on Alois's small government pension. She worked extremely hard to raise her children and managed to keep them tidily dressed and reasonably well fed.

Bloch estimated the family could afford meat no more than twice a week, providing some understanding as to why later in Hitler's life he did not feel the need to regularly consume meat, as was customary in Austria. From his mother Adolf obtained his ability to present a charming social demeanor that would later serve him well as a politician.

The most poignant aspect of Bloch's story dealt with Klara's terminal cancer and, following her death, Adolf's extensive grieving. During the fall of 1907, Klara's health deteriorated, and she died on December 21. Dr. Bloch described the intense grief Adolf suffered, attesting to the particularly close relationship between mother and son.

For Adolf, who made friends with difficulty, his mother may have been the only person he wholeheartedly loved. He had enjoyed a privileged and nearly exclusive relationship with his mother, given the early deaths of four of her other children and the seven-year age gap between Adolf and his younger sister, Paula. Klara had doted on him excessively as a young child and had been an overly permissive parent. Adolf never again gained a similar relationship that provided him such succor and devotion as that which he enjoyed with his mother.

PERFORMANCE IN SCHOOL AND BEHAVIORAL ISSUES

A child's developing personality becomes more obvious on reaching school age when he begins to mingle with other children and teachers, and so it was for young

Adolf. He had acceptable performance in his small country elementary school, but Adolf's middle school academics were poor. Certainly, Adolf was no *wunderkind*.

In his first year of Realschule, he failed both mathematics and natural history and earned low marks for conduct and diligence. Adolf failed the grade and had to repeat it. He again failed mathematics in the second level of middle school and received low scores once again for his conduct and diligence. Adolf failed French in the third year but eventually was able to pass a make-up examination.

Young Adolf was lazy in school, attending class only when he wanted to do so. His overly indulgent mother abetted his truancy, even to the extent that she allowed him to take a school year off. He then spent time in the countryside for his supposed lung ailment.

During his middle school years, one of Adolf's principal teachers, Eduard Huemer, commented in a student evaluation on Adolf's performance and especially on his prominent stubbornness. While he readily acknowledged Adolf's talent for drawing, Huemer also described Adolf's inconsiderateness, self-righteousness, and tendency toward rage. He further described Adolf's lack of self-discipline, cantankerous nature, willfulness, arrogance, and bad temper. Clearly Adolf had problems when it came to his deportment, and he had trouble fitting into the school setting. Of interest, even at this early stage of Adolf's life, his teacher noted that Adolf demanded his fellow students give their unqualified subservience to him and that Adolf imagined himself to be a leader. These personality characteristics manifested early and continued throughout his lifetime.

Psychiatrists have debated whether Hitler had developed a definable personality disorder; a lack of consensus exists regarding a specific diagnosis. However, psychologists and psychiatrists have utilized the following personality descriptors to characterize him: narcissistic, grandiose, antisocial, sociopathic, psychopathic, borderline personality, neurotic, and even delusional. These characteristics overlap with specific personality disorders, making Hitler's unusual personality difficult to pigeonhole.

Leonard Heston, a neuropsychiatrist, denies psychiatric delusions (this would in psychiatric terminology indicate psychotic thought processes), but acknowledged the more general usage of this word, meaning to hold false beliefs. The disparity between Adolf's obvious intelligence compared to his lackadaisical performance in school suggests that prominent behavioral problems existed in the youthful Hitler.

Others such as Albert Einstein were able to overcome their early childhood failures but had not suffered the demeaning and humiliating behavior to which

Adolf had been subjected. Like Einstein, Hitler developed extra motivation from his youthful challenges to succeed in his chosen profession, but he never developed the ethical underpinnings, as did Einstein, to provide moral guidance for his life.

CHAPTER 3

ADOLF'S ADOLESCENT HEALTH

A brief overview of Adolf's early health becomes useful principally to predict how Hitler would later deal with the more substantial illnesses to which he would fall prey. Adolf's health as a youth was good overall, although his vigor was less than that of the more typical robust, red-cheeked Austrian boys.

HEALTH AS A YOUTH

As a lad Adolf was frail and not very vigorous. He suffered from chronic low energy, recurring colds, and repeated bouts of influenza. Dr. Eduard Bloch described him as neither robust nor sickly but lacking the rosy, healthy cheeks of most other children that he, a family doctor, cared for in Linz. He thought the best description of Adolf was "frail looking."

Adolf was not physically impressive in stature or physical abilities and avoided athletic competitions. He was content to read a book or spend time by himself. Throughout the rest of his life, Adolf greatly feared catching colds or influenza and maintained that he was prone to suffer from a cold for six weeks or longer. This is an extraordinary claim for a viral cold. Later in his life he went to great lengths to avoid people with colds or flu, even growing irate when someone around him showed symptoms of an infectious illness.

Adolf had no serious diseases as a child, during his time in Vienna, nor even following World War I when living in Munich. Dr. Eduard Bloch in later interviews and in his 1946 memoir, *My Patient, Hitler*, denied that Adolf suffered any serious childhood illnesses. After checking his old medical records, Dr. Bloch denied ever having treated Adolf Hitler for any serious illnesses, such as the lung disease claimed by Hitler.

Dr. Bloch also commented on the adolescent Adolf's decorum and described how polite and respectful he was. This observation by Dr. Bloch differs from the school observations and demonstrates that Adolf could appear polite and not always prone to acting out in a rebellious way.

Despite Bloch's recall of Adolf having no serious illnesses, young Adolf may have believed he experienced health problems. Adolf showed an exaggerated response to what others would have considered typical childhood sicknesses. Adolf believed he had some form of lung disease that not only justified him in taking off a year from school but later excused him from service in the Austrian army.

FAMILY MEDICAL HISTORY

Considering Hitler's family medical history helps to determine if genetic or infectious illnesses or psychologically traumatizing events existed that could have affected Adolf's mental and physical health. Adolf's father, Alois Hitler, was almost certainly an alcoholic, especially during his retirement. His drunkenness no doubt aggravated his abuse of Adolf as well as Adolf's half-brother Alois Jr.

According to Brigitte Hamann, Hitler supposedly told his attorney, Hans Frank, that even as a ten- or twelve-year-old, he had to take his drunk father home from the bar: "That was the most horrible shame I have ever felt. . . . I know what a devil alcohol is! It really was—via my father—the worst enemy of my youth."

Alcoholism in parents has a substantial negative impact on the personalities of their children, often affecting the children's ability to express feelings, emotions, or establish intimacy. According to psychiatrists who have studied Adolf, he showed some of these characteristics as a child and later as an adult. In contrast to his heavy drinking father, Adolf largely abstained from alcohol.

Children of alcoholics often harbor feelings of abandonment and have a mortal fear of losing control. As we shall see later in this volume, when Germany was losing World War II Hitler responded to this threat by taking increasingly greater control of the military decision-making and relying less on his talented General Staff. Such controlling behavior would be consistent with the behavior of children of alcoholics. Nevertheless, Hitler did not exhibit this tendency early in his career as he was able to delegate and deal well with uncertainty. Later in his career he lost these abilities. Subsequent chapters will reveal an acquired medical problem that may better explain these reductions in his ability to delegate and handle uncertainty.

Sharon Martin, author of some forty self-help books, offered support for the notion of adult children of alcoholics needing to feel in control. Living with an alcoholic, she says, is scary and unpredictable, especially as a child. Trying to

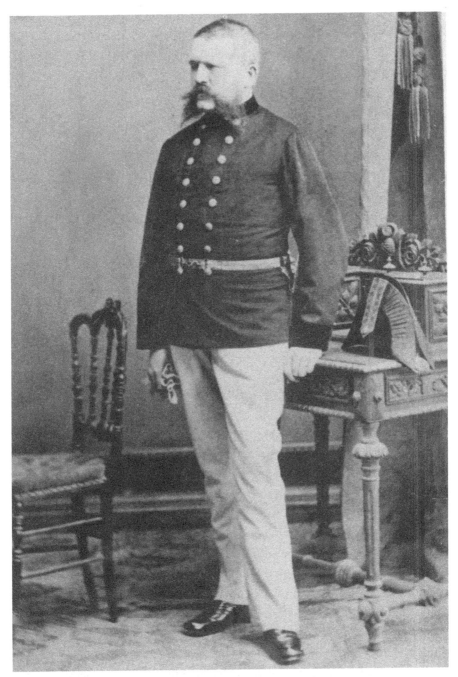

Formal portrait of Alois Hitler in his Austrian customs uniform. (Alamy stock photo)

control people is a coping strategy that children develop to deal with chaotic and dysfunctional family situations. This behavior is adaptive. Martin goes on to list characteristics as to how these control needs can show up in different ways that include the following:

Feeling uncomfortable with uncertainty.

Getting upset when things don't go your way.

Difficulty being spontaneous or having plans change.

Difficulty delegating or asking for help.

Manipulating.

Threatening or giving ultimatums.

Janet G. Woititz, in her 1983 landmark book *Adult Children of Alcoholics*, added that children of alcoholics tend to lock themselves into a course of action without giving serious consideration to alternative behaviors or to possible consequences. Some of these descriptors may sound familiar in Hitler, such as his raging when the war went against Germany, needing to be in control, and giving ultimatums. Other features sound not to be particularly descriptive of Hitler's behavior.

Soon after having taken an early medical retirement, Alois Sr. died from what was diagnosed as a pulmonary hemorrhage. Dr. Eduard Bloch inexplicably listed a cerebral hemorrhage on the death certificate (or, as he termed it, an apoplectic stroke). Death associated with a pulmonary hemorrhage in those days suggested tuberculosis, an infectious disease caused by a mycobacterium such as that which afflicted Fanny Hitler, Alois Sr.'s second wife.

Because Fanny had died of tuberculosis, the possibility exists that Alois Sr. could have contracted this infectious disease from her, and that Adolf may have been exposed to tuberculosis via his father. In those days no effective treatment existed for tuberculosis, making this illness a major killer. The largely ineffective and nonspecific treatment at that time was a healthy diet and a rest cure in the countryside.

In *Mein Kampf*, Adolf recounted how he developed a serious lung illness while attending Realschule at a time when Alois Sr. was sick enough to warrant an early medical retirement. The psychological impact of his father's dramatic death, believed to have been from a lung disease, likely stoked Adolf's own fears relating to his lung disease. Is it possible that Adolf also suffered from undiagnosed

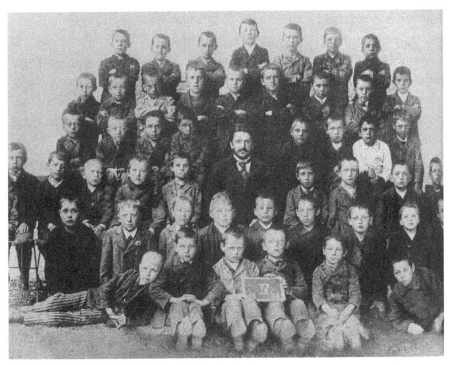

Class picture (Adolf Hitler is back row, center) in Linz, Austria, 1901. (Library of Congress, LC-USZ_61-1428; Call Number: LOT 3641)

tuberculosis contracted from his father? Since a full autopsy was not possible due to the burning of the corpse, we likely will never know for certain, but the possibility requires mentioning.

What is known is that Adolf used his lung disease as an excuse for skipping school. Klara became sufficiently concerned about Adolf's health that she arranged for him to leave school for a year and live with relatives in the countryside. Was this his rest cure for tuberculosis? Might Adolf have seen a doctor other than Dr. Eduard Bloch for diagnosis and treatment of his lung illness, thus explaining Dr. Bloch's ignorance of Adolf's pulmonary disease? Unfortunately, no medical records have been found to further explain Adolf's presumed illness.

Researchers have found no evidence that Adolf ever once in his life allowed a chest X-ray. Had a chest X-ray been taken it almost certainly would have proved or refuted a diagnosis of tuberculosis. Both for historians and his doctors, Adolf Hitler was a maddening and noncompliant patient.

In any event Adolf's pleasant sojourn in the countryside provided a welcome break from the rigors, frustrations, and failures associated with his schooling. It also provided Adolf a welcome escape from his domineering father. One wonders if, in fact, this may have been one of Klara's intentions in arranging Adolf's lengthy country holiday.

Rather than a fatal hemorrhage coming from Alois Hitler's lungs, as has been assumed, an alternative and speculative explanation exists for his death—bleeding esophageal varices. Alois Sr. could have developed alcoholic cirrhosis of the liver with the complication of esophageal varices. This liver-related illness would also have warranted the early medical retirement Alois received.

These varices are engorged veins in the esophagus and result from backpressure in the venous system due to constriction by the cirrhotic, shrunken liver. The veins in the esophagus become distended and bulge out into the central cavity of the esophagus. But these engorged varicose veins in the esophagus differ from similar varicose veins in the legs in that in the esophagus they may rupture and cause massive and often fatal bleeding. The source of the fatal hemorrhage from Alois's mouth, lacking a definitive autopsy, might have been misconstrued as originating from his lungs. In any event, witnessing or even hearing about such a horrendous sanguineous event is distressing even for experienced medical personnel and would have been psychologically devastating for a family member, especially a sensitive adolescent.

If Alois died of tuberculosis, Adolf would have been at risk for contracting this infectious disease. Alternatively, if Alois died of complications of alcoholic cirrhosis of the liver, the risk for Adolf would have been more psychological than physical. However, Adolf's recognition of his father's alcoholism and subsequent illness would be expected to impact his social habits relating to alcohol and predictably to his control needs.

As noted earlier, a psychological reaction against his alcoholic father's abusive behavior and his hatred for him may have resulted in Adolf becoming a lifelong teetotaler. Abstinence from alcohol, a known characteristic among some children of alcoholics, might also in Adolf's case be viewed as a sign of further rejection of his hated alcoholic parent.

An additional influence on Hitler's health from his FMH relates to his lifelong fear of having inherited syphilis via his father. The importance of syphilis and its potential impact for Hitler's life is deserving of its own chapter (see chapter 10).

HYPOCHONDRIASIS

Already mentioned are accounts describing young Adolf as dwelling excessively on such minor medical problems as colds and flu. Young Adolf would avoid other children for fear of illness and, if infected, would complain loudly, even if he had only acquired the sniffles.

Later in Hitler's life his doctors similarly believed many of his complaints to be psychosomatic and overwrought. The basis of his hypochondriasis began early, possibly as a mechanism to garner attention from his parents, especially from his mother and possibly as a ploy to extract sympathy from his demanding and emotionally distant father. Later in life Hitler's associates noted how he exhibited a marked fear of germs and was known to carry out compulsive hand washing to reduce his risk of infection.

Young Adolf emerged from childhood as an orphaned intelligent child, but one who had suffered emotionally and physically from an abusive and alcoholic father. Young Adolf had enjoyed a strong and protective relationship with his mother. His hatred for his father grew as he endured not only his father's wrath but also having witnessed his father's mistreatment of his beloved mother. Adolf showed great stubbornness and narcissism, was subject to giving intense but rambling orations, and wished to dominate those around him. He also developed signs of excessive rumination on his body that would later evolve into frank hypochondriasis.

CHAPTER 4

THE VIENNA PERIOD

Once children leave the protection of their immediate families, their personality characteristics become increasingly evident. So too did Adolf Hitler begin his transformation from childhood and adolescence into becoming the adult that the world would know as the man who changed the course of history in the twentieth century. A review of this period of Hitler's life helps our understanding as to how he transformed from being a polite but mischievous boy to becoming a harsh dictator. As it relates to Hitler's medical history, the Vienna period appears to have been a healthy one while his personality became crystallized.

DISAPPOINTMENT AND SHAME IN VIENNA

After being expelled from Realschule in 1904, the following year Adolf moved to Vienna. By then in his mid-teens, he lived a Bohemian existence and supported himself on a state orphan's pension (only his mother remained alive at that point) and limited financial assistance from his mother.

On arriving in Vienna, Hitler rented a small room that he felt was below his preferred standards. For a time, Adolf worked in construction where his fellow workers appeared to have disliked him. A story from Eduard Bloch relates how Adolf's co-workers once threatened to push him off a scaffold, suggesting he was far from popular on the job site. Hitler also mentioned this story in *Mein Kampf*. Whether in this instance Adolf's lack of popularity with his co-workers stemmed from his fondness for giving lectures, was due to his laziness, resulted from his prudishness, or for other reasons is not entirely clear.

Although later when he wrote *Mein Kampf* Hitler stressed his deprivation in Vienna, some authors have claimed that Adolf had a modest but reasonably carefree existence there. Brigitte Hamann described that Adolf was so poor that he spent time in a homeless shelter. One impression she shared of the twenty-year-old Hitler was that he seemed sad, was dead-tired and starved, and had sore feet. He had by then sold any possessions brought from Linz and owned only the shabby clothes that he wore. Other authors, such as Dr. Eduard Bloch, described Hitler as living in the equivalent of an American flophouse.

Bloch said Adolf's sordid surroundings and low-class companions gave rise to increasing unhappiness in Adolf. It was Bloch's assessment that this unhappiness later spread to a broader hatred of societal institutions including government and trade unions as well as foreigners. Adolf continued to employ his often-used defense mechanism of scapegoating, blaming societal ills on foreigners and Jews who had different customs and language.

Hitler spent much of his nonworking time reading newspapers, pamphlets, and publications at the public libraries and cafes. He was not a serious reader nor was he a deep thinker. Hitler showed a fondness for German hero mythology and military topics. He came to believe simplistically that world history could be reduced to a struggle between superior blond-haired, blue-eyed Aryans and ape-like, inferior populations.

Fritz Redlich stated in his psychiatrically oriented study that Hitler was an ardent German nationalist with strong ethnophobic beliefs. Hitler disregarded the experiences of the people in Vienna whom he viewed as non-German, particularly Czechs and Jews. He also believed that whether other countries loved Germany was immaterial—it was only important that they feared Germany.

Hitler enjoyed reading fiction. He particularly liked James Fennimore Cooper's writings. Cooper had written a series of historical romances of frontier and American Indian life. Hitler was also especially fond of the highly fictionalized western novels written by the German author Karl May. May had never placed his German foot on American soil, nor had he ever met a Native American. It can truly be said of May that he never let the facts get in the way of a good story. Various authors have claimed Karl May was one of the major, but inaccurate, influences on Hitler and that it may have underpinned Hitler's understanding of the taming of the American West.

Speculation exists that the near eradication of Native Americans and the forced removal of the remaining subjugated tribes onto reservations may have become a political construct that Hitler internalized and later repeated when incarcerating Jews and other perceived undesirables. Hitler is believed to have viewed this approach as civilized Europeans rightfully subduing the inferior peoples of the world, the *Untermenschen*. Adolf also incorporated the prevalent colonial and anti-Semitic narratives of the time into his worldview.

Hitler never traveled extensively. His knowledge of other cultures, languages, and environments was quite limited. His meager income may in part explain his lack of travel. Even more, Hitler's lack of interest in or respect for other cultures was present and was apparent to those who interacted with him.

As noted earlier, Hitler's grandiosity became evident during his childhood when he drew plans to redo his hometown of Linz and make it into a magnificent city. This trait in Adolf became even more apparent while he was living in Vienna. He began to write plays and at one point even attempted to bring one of Wagner's unpublished works to the stage. He tackled the Wagner challenge with stupendous energy, even cajoling his friend, August Kubizek, to assist in this nearly impossible effort. Later Adolf abandoned his quest when he was unable to make any serious headway.

In Vienna, Adolf vehemently disliked the many foreign students and others from far-flung areas of the Austro-Hungarian Empire. He thought of these groups as culturally, ethnically, and otherwise inferior to native Germans. Austria's sense of national pride and chagrin at being part of a fading empire coupled with his father's influence of intolerance may have encouraged his disdain for foreigners.

Hitler became painfully aware of Jews who were in control of large banks. He also found Jews to be numerous throughout the arts and professions. Adolf came to believe their presence in such high positions of power and influence prevented Aryans from assuming their rightful and prominent roles in society. He felt foreigners were stealing the jobs that should have gone to Austrians or Germans. His long-repressed anger targeted them with his hatred.

Both in 1907 and 1908, Adolf applied to the Vienna Academy of Fine Arts, but both times the Academy rejected his application. Gaining entrance to the Academy was, after all, the very reason Adolf had set off for Vienna to improve his talents as a visual artist. He was thunderstruck by the rejections. Recall his long desire to become an artist and the many arguments with his father over his choice of vocation. The fact that only twenty-eight out of 113 candidates were accepted into the painting school according to Hamann offered little consolation to the suffering Adolf.

According to John Toland, August Kubizek learned of Adolf's searing disappointment and rejection when Adolf gave a bitter denunciation of the Academy of Fine Arts by describing the faculty as "a lot of old-fashioned fossilized civil servants, bureaucrats, devoid of understanding, stupid lumps of officials. The whole Academy ought to be blown up!"

In Vienna, Adolf's great ambition to become an artist was shattered. The Academy unceremoniously cited "unfitness for painting" and advised Adolf to

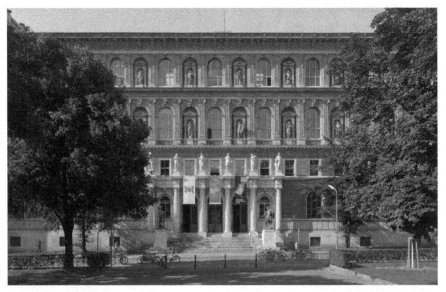

Vienna Academy of Fine Arts, where Adolf was denied admission. (Peter Hass / CC BY-SA 3.0)

seek training in architecture. To add to his misery, his lack of a diploma from Realschule and not having the necessary preparation from the required Technical School prevented him from applying for entrance to the architecture school. At that point Adolf's vocational aspirations had hit a galling dead end.

Many students at the Institute of Art and at the Institute of Architecture hailed from outlying areas of the Austro-Hungarian Empire. The presence of the enrolled foreign students infuriated the young and xenophobic Hitler. Here were people who had bested him by gaining admission to these two institutes for the training he so desperately sought and thought he deserved. This travesty, as he likely viewed it, is believed to have further developed his hatred and distrust of foreigners.

It was during this period of educational humiliation in Vienna that Adolf's beloved mother died following her struggle with breast cancer. This crushing loss further exacerbated Adolf's melancholy and removed his main source of affection and a portion of his financial support. To make matters still worse, a court in Linz ordered him to turn over his orphan's benefits to his sister, Paula. Some accounts claim Adolf voluntarily gave up his portion of the pension to his younger sister. In any event, even greater financial desperation then stalked the grieving and brooding young Adolf.

To survive, the desperate Adolf began copying scenes from postcards and hawking them to tourists. During this financially and emotionally distraught period of his life, Adolf was orphaned, penurious, and as adrift as a rudderless, flat-bottomed Zille (boat) on the Danube.

DEVELOPMENT OF HITLER'S ANTI-SEMITISM

Hitler claimed in *Mein Kampf* that it was during this developmental phase of his life in Vienna that he became an anti-Semite. This was after all the first time in Adolf's life that he had contact with any substantial number of Jews. His loss of his mother, his failure as an artist, and his penury would have acted as psychological stressors and would have magnified his psychological defense of scapegoating.

A source of Hitler's developing anti-Semitism has been thought to originate from the many Jewish administrators and professors at the Vienna Academy of Fine Arts. According to Brigitte Hamann, however, none of the four professors who directly refused Adolf's admission were Jewish. She claimed that any such speculation was entirely unfounded.

Considering Adolf's longing to create art, this huge personal disappointment and blow to his ego would have strained his ability psychologically to cope. Given the large number of Jewish students and faculty (as well as the numerous Slavic students from the far-flung Austro-Hungarian Empire) at the Institute of Art, this Jewish and Slavic influence arguably may have mobilized Hitler's tendency to scapegoat.

Adolf's anguishes in Vienna rose at an alarming rate. His pain and rage built to enormous levels, and he dealt with his psychological woes immaturely. His perorations to his friend Kubizek took on new vehemence. His hatred for Jews firmly took hold along with contempt for those who were not ethnic Austrian or German. His practice of scapegoating his anger and frustrations steadily grew into frank xenophobia and anti-Semitism.

Hitler's reaction to the death of his mother Klara proved revealing. Aspects of her care, according to Rudolph Binion in his 1976 book *Hitler among the Germans*, possibly contributed to Adolf's growing anti-Semitism. In the winter of 1906–1907, Klara Hitler became very ill. Dr. Eduard Bloch, a Jewish general physician, diagnosed her as having breast cancer. Klara underwent surgery performed by Dr. Karl Urban at a local hospital. Dr. Bloch continued to treat Klara post-operatively for an infected chest wound by repeatedly packing the surgical wound with iodoform gauze.

Binion concluded that Hitler's anti-Semitism might have deepened from his conviction that the Jewish Dr. Bloch had mistreated his mother by excessive use of iodoform gauze, had failed to relieve her pain (German general practitioners at the time were not allowed to inject morphine), and had financially exploited his family. It is difficult to understand medically why packing a wound with iodoform gauze would lead to any serious side effects. Certainly, scapegoating by a young and inexperienced young man, prostrate with grief, remains a possibility. Failure to relieve pain is more difficult to assess. Only limited pain management strategies existed for Bloch, and Klara likely suffered greatly from her widely metastatic breast cancer. This condition would have been agonizing, not only for Klara, but also emotionally for Adolf and the rest of her family.

Author Fritz Redlich drew different conclusions regarding the relationship between Bloch and Hitler. Based on Hitler's 1938 grateful references to Dr. Bloch and his recognition of his mother's poor prognosis from the outset, many doubt Bloch played a major role in ramping up Hitler's anti-Semitism. In support of this latter view, Hitler sent two personally drawn postcards from Vienna to Bloch. Dr. Bloch described one of these cards:

> It showed a hooded Capuchin monk hoisting a glass of bubbling champagne. Under the picture was a caption: "Prosit Neujahr—a toast to the New Year." On the reverse side he had written a message: "The Hitler family sends you the best wishes for a Happy New Year. In everlasting thankfulness, Adolf Hitler."

Years later the Gestapo appeared at Bloch's home, requesting first to view and then to appropriate the two postcards. The officer scribbled a receipt for the two postcards, one of which had been hand drawn by Adolf Hitler. An agent by the name of Groemer signed the receipt and told Dr. Bloch and his wife to come to headquarters the following morning. The next day the agent in charge, when learning of Dr. Bloch's Jewishness, grew distant and informed Bloch that the postcards would be maintained for safekeeping.

Nevertheless, the Gestapo acted with uncharacteristic courtesy toward the Jewish Dr. Bloch. Such a friendly act as sending hand-painted postcards to Dr. Bloch would be surprising if Hitler had disliked the physician. No doubt because of Hitler's intervention the Gestapo acted far more gingerly than was their customary behavior toward Jews.

Dr. Bloch's possession of these gifts could have led to embarrassment for Hitler, especially given the Nuremberg Laws that denied Jews German citizenship or the right to fly the German flag. In addition, because of Hitler's intervention Dr. Bloch was allowed to continue his medical practice in Linz but eventually had to limit it to treating only Jews. Dr. Bloch also did not have to mark his home in yellow paint, wear a marker identifying him as Jewish, surrender his passport, or have his ration card stamped with the letter "J."

The ration card without the "J" allowed Bloch to shop at any time, whereas ration cards marked with the "J" were limited to inconvenient shopping times when goods were largely picked over. Eventually Bloch was permitted to sell his home at market prices and emigrate to the United States. Hitler had referred to his family doctor as an *Edeljude* or "noble Jew" and said that if all Jews were like him, Germany would not have a Jewish problem. Hitler's kind acts toward Dr. Bloch certainly do not support Binion's suggestion that poor medical treatment by Dr. Bloch underscored or increased Hitler's anti-Semitism.

It was in Vienna that Adolf began developing rigidly held views that Jews were the enemies of Aryans, and that they had caused Austria's political and economic crisis. He blamed Jews such as Karl Marx and Leon Trotsky for having played principal roles in developing and promoting communism, a political philosophy he thoroughly detested.

In *Mein Kampf* Adolf Hitler explained how in Vienna his anti-Semitism had grown:

> Since I had begun to concern myself with this question and to take cognizance of the Jews, Vienna appeared to me in a different light than before. Wherever I went, I began to see Jews, and the more I saw, the more sharply they became distinguished in my eyes from the rest of humanity. Particularly the Inner City and the districts north of the Danube Canal swarmed with a people that even outwardly had lost all resemblance to Germans...
>
> All this could scarcely be called very attractive; but it became positively repulsive when, in addition to their physical uncleanliness, you discovered the moral stains on this "chosen people"...
>
> Was there any form of filth or profligacy, particularly in cultural life, without at least one Jew involved in it?
>
> If you cut even cautiously into such an abscess, you found, like a maggot in a rotting body, often dazzled by the sudden light—a kike!
>
> Gradually I began to hate them.

Hitler later came to believe that Jewish involvement had led to Germany's defeat in World War I. Eduard Bloch, his Jewish family physician, affirmed Hitler's timing of his acquiring such anti-Jewish bias by saying that in Linz the youth he knew was not an anti-Semite, but that he had picked up this trait while living in Vienna. By the conclusion of the Vienna period, Adolf Hitler's personality showed growing anti-Semitism and was marbled with extreme stubbornness, egoism, grandiosity, a penchant for oratory, and cruelty.

CHAPTER 5

WORLD WAR I

The onset of World War I would stoke Hitler's pan-German nationalism and introduce him to military life. Both developments provided him a sense of belonging to something greater than himself. Hitler suffered physical injuries during World War I that provide insights into his assessment of himself and into his mental health. This portion of his social history also proves important for establishing his life's ambitions and providing goals and meaning for his life.

MILITARY SERVICE

When World War I threatened, Adolf claimed his old "severe pulmonary disease" to avoid service in the Austrian army. A medical determination made in Salzburg found Hitler "too weak to bear arms" in the Austrian military. Hitler's "frail appearance" as Dr. Eduard Bloch had once described and Hitler's claim of a past lung condition saved him from conscription into the Austrian army.

However, on August 10, 1914, Hitler did not hesitate to join the German Sixteenth Bavarian Reserve Infantry Regiment (often referred to as the List Regiment) where he was made a private. During his service he appeared an ardent German nationalist, even though Austrian by birth.

It may seem strange by today's standards for Hitler to have become such a German nationalist since he was Austrian, but it bears remembering that Austria had been part of the Holy Roman Empire that included many German states. Austria was also part of the German Confederation until the Austro-Prussian War in 1866. Hitler often harkened back to a recollection of this pan-German state, and he became an ardent supporter of Georg von Schönerer's Pan-German Party in Austria. This political party appealed to the German elements in the multinational Austrian empire to protect their allegedly threatened ethnicity against the rising demands of Slavic peoples. Later in Hitler's life, creating such a pan-German state became his overriding goal.

Hitler's decision to join a German regiment along with his contemptuousness for the decrepit, multinational Habsburg Empire can also be viewed psychologically as a jab at his father, the quintessentially proud Austrian. Had Alois Hitler lived, Adolf's decision to serve in the German Army, rather than the Austrian army, no doubt would have provoked Alois's stern rebuke.

Biographer Joachim Fest in his 1968 book *Hitler* argued that World War I made all the difference in Hitler's radicalization. Before the war, Hitler had been a lazy artist with poorly directed ambition. Following the war, Hitler was determined to save Germany from its defeat and reestablish it as a great nation. The time Hitler spent in World War I while serving in the List Regiment is believed to have shaped his subsequent personality and life's work. Thomas Weber attempted in his 2017 book *Becoming Hitler: The Making of a Nazi* to explain this transformation, not based on the sparse records of Hitler himself but on the activities of the List Regiment in which Hitler served.

In the German Army, Adolf rose to the rank of corporal. He received both an Iron Cross, second class, and an Iron Cross, first class, that underscored his demonstrated bravery, earning these military decorations by running messages under fire between German frontline positions and headquarters. His dispatch-running service was dangerous work and carried out under perilous conditions with bullets flying overhead. Thomas Weber in his book *Hitler's First War* (2011) tends to downplay any unusual bravery on the part of Hitler given that all four of the dispatch runners for the regiment won Iron Crosses. Weber argues that the decoration typically went to officers or enlisted men who were well known to their commanding officers. Since Hitler worked out of regimental headquarters, he was known by those making up the awards list. The significance of his being awarded an Iron Cross, as it pertains to his bravery, has remained controversial.

Undoubtedly, during his time as a dispatch runner, Hitler must have witnessed mutilated bodies lying on blood-soaked battlefields. The stench of death, choking smoke, destroyed military equipment, dead animals, and pervasive agony of wounded and dying soldiers would seemingly have impacted him, as such horror did other soldiers on both sides of the conflict. Nevertheless, no reports are available of Hitler's emotional response, if any, to such human carnage and tragedy. While we have no such descriptions by Hitler, others in the List Regiment gave descriptions, according to Weber, of squeezing by dead bodies and comrades with ghastly injuries. Whether Hitler's lack of emotional response to the carnage of warfare

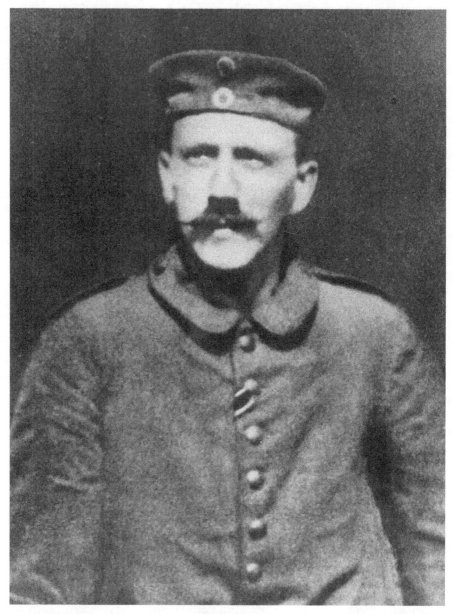

Corporal Hitler, World War I. (Alamy stock photo)

and death of comrades is an artifact of missing history or whether the absence of his emotional empathizing is a feature of his personality remains arguable.

According to Fritz Redlich, Adolf's fellow soldiers, while respecting him for his bravery, described him as aloof, doctrinaire, prudish, and eccentric. By running dispatches between headquarters and the trenches, Hitler managed to gain insights into military tactics and strategy that typical trench-bound infantrymen did not have access to. Hitler's job also provided him with an unusual amount of autonomy that fit him well, being the loner that he was.

Nevertheless, World War I according to Weber did not make Hitler the Nazi he became. Contrary to Nazi propaganda, Hitler oscillated between various left-wing and right-wing socialist ideas and showed no animosity to the Jewish soldiers in his unit. His experience in the List Regiment seems not to have heightened his anti-Semitism. Hitler clearly had developed his dislike for the international world and believed that the war would smash not only external enemies but also internal ones that espoused internationalism. For Hitler achieving this nationalist goal made the terrible cost of the war worthwhile. Also, despite what the Nazi propagandists later espoused, Hitler was not particularly well thought of by his fellow soldiers, even being referred to as *Etappenschweiner* (literally rear-echelon pigs) due to his supposed cushy lifestyle a few miles behind the front lines.

HITLER INJURED

At the Battle of the Somme on October 5, 1916, Adolf received a shell fragment to his left thigh. According to Weber a British small grenade hit just at the front entrance of the dispatch runners' rear line dugout. Hitler, along with fellow dispatch runners Anton Bachmann and Ernst Schmidt, was wounded. His wound was slight according to the official Bavarian casualty list but proved serious enough to have Hitler sent home.

Hitler would later claim this wound became a source of chronic discomfort, although his scar would later disappear. Hitler and Nazi propaganda repeatedly embellished the degree of Hitler's wound and the circumstances under which he acquired it. Hitler's political gain from having sustained a war wound and his lifelong overemphasis of his symptoms suggest his residual shrapnel wound's afflictions were minimal or nonexistent.

Hitler's other more serious war injury occurred on October 14, 1918, when he was partially blinded in an English mustard gas attack. John Toland in the first volume of his 1976 work *Adolf Hitler* provides an enlightening description of the events as follows:

> During October of 1918 the 16th Bavarian Reserve Infantry Regiment in which Hitler served came under a devastating British artillery attack. The assault consisted of artillery shells pounding the lines of the dispirited German lines. On the night of the 13th of October in addition to the artillery shells falling came a lethal assault by mustard gas

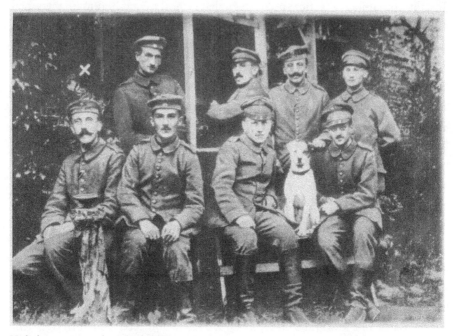

Hitler's army comrades, who held him in low esteem, during World War I. Adolf is in the front row, on the left. (United States National Archives. Record Group 208, NA identifier 535934, Local identifier 208-FU-93Y (4))

shelling. A pungent cloud of mustard gas spread over the German positions, killing some troops and sending the remaining troops scrambling for their gas masks. It was dawn before the mustard gas began to dissipate but shortly following the sunrise the mustard gas shelling resumed. Virtually all the German troops were blinded in the attacks. One soldier who had some remaining sight called for his fellow soldiers to form a line and hold onto the man in front of him. This soldier led the blinded soldiers away from the battlefield and toward the train that would take them to various hospitals.

Shortly thereafter, Hitler reported for treatment at the Neurology and Psychiatry department of the reserve hospital at Pasewalk. The mustard gas caused his eyes to burn terribly, the mucous membranes to become inflamed, and his eyelids and face to swell. In response to the injury, Adolf's eye closure muscles went into spasm, forcing his eyes shut.

A threatened loss of vision would be a catastrophe for anyone, but even more so for Hitler, given his artistic leanings. No doubt his eye injury was both painful and psychologically threatening.

Over several weeks, his eyesight slowly returned. Then on November 10, 1918, a strange phenomenon occurred when Hitler suffered a relapse. The timing of the relapse elicited suspicion and incredulousness on the part of his treating physicians. It seemed his relapse immediately followed his learning that Germany had surrendered to the Western Allies and that the German emperor had abdicated. This second loss of vision brought about another round of medical assessment.

According to John Toland and Rudolph Binion, Hitler then received treatment from a consulting psychiatrist, Professor Edmund Forster, the chief of the Berlin University Nerve Clinic. Forster believed Hitler's sudden relapse represented an episode of hysteria. Forster established this purely psychological diagnosis, as he could find no medical reason for the recurring visual loss. Forster also believed Hitler was a psychopath (lacking any conscience for the suffering of others) in addition to demonstrating hysterical (purely psychologically caused) symptoms.

Robert Waite, in his 1977 book *The Psychopathic God Adolf Hitler*, takes issue with the conclusions of Toland and Binion regarding their sources since no paperwork from the hospital in Pasewalk could be located to document the psychiatric diagnosis and treatment. Waite says these records, if they ever existed, were destroyed perhaps at the later direction of Hitler.

PLANTING SEEDS OF REPRESSED ANGER

A foundation is required for understanding Forster's diagnosis of hysteria. By various accounts Hitler had been mortified on learning of Germany's defeat. This catastrophic event created in him a tremendous sense of rage, rage that he was unable to dissipate or address in a psychologically healthy manner. Such unresolved emotional turmoil is believed to be at the core of hysterical illnesses.

Immediately after learning of Germany's defeat, Hitler stormed back to his bed and covered his head with his pillow and blankets. He lay there stewing in his anger, his profound disappointment fueling his desire to somehow change or deny Germany's defeat. It was then that he again lost his vision.

Hitler along with many of his comrades in arms believed the German leaders had effectively stabbed them and their country in the back. They saw this surrender as a betrayal of its brave soldiers. As he had learned to do earlier in his life, Hitler then sought a convenient scapegoat. He focused on Jews and blamed them for Germany's defeat, ascribing their motive to monetary gains.

Blaming the Jews for social catastrophes, such as downturns in the economy, was nothing new in German history. During the stock market crash of 1873, a dramatic increase in anti-Semitism occurred. Many Jews at the time were employed in finance and banking. Due to anti-Semitism in earlier times, these professions were some of the few available to them. Jews collectively were blamed for the "speculation fever" that led up to the stock market crash.

Also, Hitler along with many comrades in World War I believed their German leaders had negotiated badly, that they had accepted defeat far too easily, and that the sacrifices of Germany's brave soldiers had been for naught. Hitler's deep-seated anger continued to smolder over time such that it would later fire his political activism and morph into another conflagration.

As Hitler lay on his cot, sensing profound despair and rage, he felt as if life had become unbearable. It was then that he states he experienced a supernatural experience. Hitler heard a voice urging him to save Germany. Some writers claim this voice was that of the Virgin Mary. Hitler described to intimates that as the miracle came to pass the darkness that had eclipsed his vision suddenly disappeared. It was then that Hitler made a vow that he would devote his life's entire energies to carrying out this command to save Germany from further treachery.

Some speculation exists that Professor Forster might have induced the hallucination through drugs, although no medical records exist to prove or disprove this conjecture. That day in Pasewalk, Hitler experienced a sudden, lucid awareness of his life's calling that would animate this command to save Germany. This mysticism would later propel the world to the razor edge of utter destruction.

As a neurologist, many times I have witnessed similar patient recoveries in those with conversion reactions (hysteria). At a time when the symptoms appear no longer psychologically helpful or supportive to the patient's psychological needs, an intervention—consisting of a presumed treatment—usually brings about a dramatic and complete recovery. For example, patients with hysterical walking problems or paralysis of limbs or visual loss might be left with the therapeutic suggestion that their malady would require placement in some unwished-for long-term facility. Such a suggestion removes whatever psychological benefits (gain) the hysterical loss has contributed.

At this juncture the administration of a so-called Black Box treatment such as minimal electrical stimulation or other faux treatment, such as infusion of a benign medication with strong psychological suggestion of a cure, will oftentimes "cure" the patient. In Hitler's case Dr. Forster may have so acted and provided Hitler a face-saving way to get rid of his hysterical blindness.

Despite complete recovery from his visual loss, Hitler, after the war, would still refer to himself as a blinded cripple. The issue of hysteria (believed to be a subconscious effect of which the patient is unaware) or malingering (faking a symptom or illness) has been considered by medical historians in Hitler's case, yet little definitive proof exists. Conveniently, Hitler's medical records from the hospital at Pasewalk disappeared.

It is of interest that Adolf Hitler was hospitalized in a Neurology and Psychiatry facility, rather than in a general medical facility. This choice of facility suggests the possibility that at the outset the medical team may have suspected hysteria or malingering. Alternatively, the large number of wounded may simply have overwhelmed all other available general medical facilities and required usage of all remaining beds.

Hysteria or conversion reaction, the latter term being common reference today, most frequently exists in psychologically unsophisticated individuals with limited education and poor psychological insight. Typically, such patients view life in black and white terms. This description fits Hitler well, both as a patient and for his relapse.

Some caution here is needed. Undoubtedly hysteria in the early twentieth century was over-diagnosed. This was due to limited understanding of neurological disorders at the time. But Hitler's medically unexplainable total visual relapse under those circumstances strongly suggests a diagnosis of conversion reaction.

Toland further recounts Hitler's unusual delusion or vision that had directed him to save Germany. According to Toland this apparition makes Hitler sound like a prophet from the Old Testament, and certainly his deep-seated conviction that followed could have inspired his political ambition. While Hitler later embraced his perceived role as the savior of Germany, he wisely distanced himself from his prophetic apparition, as the German people would have viewed this skeptically, even derisively.

Mustard gas gives rise to severe irritation to the skin and especially to the sensitive membranes of the eyes. It causes inflammation of the eyes and light sensitivity and leads to swelling that was extreme enough to close Hitler's eyes. It caused the muscles of his eyes to spasm, forcing his eyes to close (the medical term is blepharospasm). But mustard gas does not cause relapses. Parenthetically, it also does not increase the risk for Parkinson's disease or heart disease, two major illnesses from which Hitler would later suffer.

Hitler's experience in the German Army during World War I had one more major social impact on his life. Hitler for the first time experienced a welcome sense of belonging to an entity larger than himself. This portion of Hitler's social history is significant in that Adolf had few friends as a child or while living in Vienna. The army had provided him a sense of community and a sense of purpose that gave newfound meaning to his life.

Given his harangues, standoffishness, and prudishness (he disliked the bawdy humor of the other soldiers), Hitler was far from the most popular person in his unit. Nevertheless, the opinion among officers and enlisted men alike was that Hitler acted courageously and constituted an able soldier. Despite Hitler's bravery, he was not promoted beyond corporal. Arguably in one of the greatest errors in leadership assessment in history, Hitler was said to lack leadership abilities.

An attitude of companionship and solidarity existed among the largely trench-bound troops, making Hitler feel, perhaps for one of the few times in his early life, needed and appreciated. Even more importantly Hitler, who had lost his last parent as a teenager and who had failed as an artist, had finally found a position where his drive and courage could be put on full display. The List Regiment had become his new home and something of a parent to him; as will be seen, Hitler would prove reluctant to give up his newfound sense of belonging.

CHAPTER 6

BECOMING HITLER IN MUNICH

With the drama and human suffering of World War I behind him, Adolf Hitler struck out to further define himself in Munich. As is expected at this stage of a person's life, Hitler's personality characteristics became still better established. These features along with the political and cultural events of the time were to shape the contours of his life. His social experiences in Munich helped to form the adult Adolf Hitler and to provide the capacity and associations that led him on his meteoric rise to become *der Führer*.

The dramatic cultural shifts in Western civilization that occurred in the early twentieth century provided a backdrop upon which Hitler's maturation unfolded. At the time Christianity was under assault. It had always been the prevailing force that provided meaning to the lives of people. Science and pseudoscience held increasing sway, and people struggled to find meaning in their difficult industrialized lives. Open class warfare existed. The Austro-Hungarian Empire was imploding, and a flood of refugees sought sanctuary in Western Europe. These immigrant migrations caused additional cultural friction and societal confusion.

Following World War I, the harsh terms meted out by the victorious Allies brought about an increase in German poverty and stoked anger among the defeated and fearful German populace. The main terms of the Treaty of Versailles were reparations to the Allied powers in the staggering amount of five billion dollars and required Germany to disarm and give up its colonies.

The onset of the Great Depression further battered world economies, causing still greater personal suffering and deprivation in a defeated Germany. Germany suffered substantially because of its loans being recalled by the United States.

This financial blow caused its economy to collapse and sent poverty soaring. The Treaty of Versailles planted toxic seeds that later stoked Germany's humiliation and resentment. It was in this chaos and societal suffering that the mature Adolf Hitler first strode forth upon the world stage.

POSTWAR MUNICH

Following his recovery from the mustard gas attack near the conclusion of World War I, Hitler had no real home or family to which to return. He was rapidly mustered out of his unit. The practical consideration confronting him was that he needed a place to live and a job to support himself. Hitler decided to move to Munich in Bavaria, a region of Germany which he knew well.

As elsewhere in Germany following the war, Hitler found Munich a chaotic, teeming environment. Emperor Wilhelm II had fled the country and a socialist, Friedrich Ebert, had become the president of the newly established Weimar Republic. A series of leaders emerged but were overthrown either through assassination or resignation. The Weimar Republic was a bourgeois government that enjoyed the support of the German Army.

The communists led frequent but poorly organized marches, preaching that the international workers should arise and rid themselves of the shackles of the bourgeoisie. The communists called openly for class warfare.

Riots broke out in Munich between the revolutionary communists and the counterrevolutionary ex-soldiers and nationalists. The latter group was largely composed of veterans of military service in World War I and who greatly respected authority, desired discipline, and distrusted international influences. Given this toxic stew of political philosophies, it is not surprising that open conflict arose, and killings occurred. The government and the army struggled to suppress these revolutionary and counterrevolutionary groups.

During this dramatic hinge of history, Hitler lived in strife-torn Munich with his developing but fluctuating political convictions, seeking direction and purpose for his life.

NEW HORIZONS

Hitler managed to find a job with the Press and News Bureau of the Political Department of the German Army's Munich Command. He underwent a course in political instruction and was assigned the task of preventing the spread of such alien ideas as socialism and pacifism. He must have welcomed such an assignment to support a nationalistic German government.

For suppressing the many uprisings, the Weimar Republic dispatched army units throughout Germany. The weak Weimar government sought intelligence regarding ongoing revolutionary developments so that the impact of these movements could be quelled quickly. While Hitler had some misgivings about the Weimar government given its embrace of the upper classes, he so disliked the communists and Jews that he was happy to be recruited to spy on the various revolutionary groups in Munich.

In September 1919, Hitler was directed to investigate the affairs of a small political group, the German Workers' Party. A locksmith, Anton Drexler, had organized the party in 1916. Drexler had wished to create a party that was both nationalistic and working class. According to a report conducted after Hitler's death by Morris Leikind in 1945 (not fully released until 2000), only a few workers at the time attended the meetings of this new political party. Despite the small size of the party, it would afford Hitler a great organizational opportunity.

Hitler attended political meetings that were held mostly in Munich beer halls. He would file reports on the various revolutionary groups, describe risks for unwanted political activities, and report on any political goals unpopular with the existing government.

After attending a host of meetings of the German Workers' Party, Hitler developed a distinct affinity for their ideals, as they closely matched his own growing convictions. These objectives included removal of the strict class structure in Germany and creation of a unified pan-German state (usually referred to as a Greater Germany or German Empire). Their slogan was "Common Good Above Individual Good." The German Workers' Party did not recognize the right of Jews to be German citizens. It also practiced misogyny and had no consideration for women in prominent party positions. The party also was hostile to the Treaty of Versailles and its stiff financial penalties on Germany. These goals resonated with the nationalistic, anti-Semitic, xenophobic, misogynistic, socialist that Adolf Hitler had by then become.

The small group of German Workers' Party supporters frequently met in the back room of a Munich beer hall. Hitler became progressively attracted by their desire for a pan-German state and by their profound anti-Semitism. After a time, Hitler stopped filing his reports on this group and became inexorably drawn more and more into the workings of this small political party.

On February 24, 1920, the German Workers' Party changed its name to the National Socialist German Workers' Party (NSDAP) or as it more commonly has been referred to as the Nazi Party. Hitler's remarkable oratorical skills had

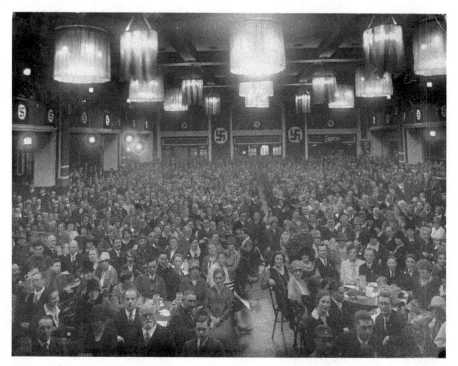

Meeting of the NSDAP in the Bürgerbräukeller, Munich, 1923. (Bundesarchiv Bild 146-1978-004-12A)

by then become apparent. His effective oratory along with his recruitment abilities prompted both growth of the party's membership and his rapid rise within the party's leadership. Largely due to Hitler's influence, the party prospered. It began to attract various splinter political groups from Austria and the Sudetenland. It became progressively more anti-Semitic and began to use the *Hakenkreuz*—the swastika—as its symbol.

During his climb through the ranks of the party, Hitler came to believe that the spoken word was more convincing and would recruit more people than would the written word. He thought oratory had been greatly beneficial for all the prominent political movements of history. Hitler's belief may have defaulted from his own relative inability to write a coherent sentence in stark contrast to his remarkable oratorical skills. Clearly Adolf Hitler was a persuasive orator but not a very good writer. Hitler's speeches lengthened and became progressively more impassioned. To be sure, Hitler's appeal to the people stemmed from his boundless energy, his frenzied oratory, and his emotionality—not from his grasp of history, economics, critical thinking, or careful reasoning.

He began to draw progressively larger audiences to the National Socialist Workers' Party. Hitler's beliefs and oratorical skills launched his political identity and over the next decade would power his meteoric career path that eventually led him to become the chancellor of Germany.

With consummate energy Hitler immersed himself in heady political issues. As described by Thomas Weber in *Becoming Hitler*, he showed considerable political skills, elbowing his way into leadership positions. When sounded out about serving as chairman of the propaganda committee, Hitler leapt at the opportunity. But it was Hitler's well-practiced oratorical skills developed in the back room of a beer garden in revolutionary Munich that would later enable him to mesmerize a war-weary Germany to mobilize for war. While controversy exists regarding the extent of Hitler's wartime leadership skills, no doubt exists regarding his leadership abilities when it came to organizing and energizing a political movement.

Hitler developed a pattern for his speech making. Oftentimes he would initially stand at the lectern saying nothing for several minutes. He would then begin his presentations with soft tones and measured pauses. Then during the speech, he progressively would work himself into a frenzied state such that by the end of the speech Hitler was haranguing his audience at the top of his lungs.

Hitler's style of oratory proved remarkably effective. As he had done years before with his childhood friend August Kubizek, Hitler was able to capture the emotions of his audiences, but his style of oratory was not without personal sacrifice. Even early in his life, Hitler had one recurring voice-related medical problem correlating to his manner of oratory. For anyone who has listened to Hitler's speeches, it is easy to understand how his screaming, over-the-top speechmaking could lead to hoarseness, vocal cord damage, and vocal cord polyps.

On several occasions later in life, the polyps required surgical removal under cocaine analgesia. After each treatment, as will be described in a later chapter, his symptoms would improve, but not before he had also developed a fondness for cocaine.

THE HITLER MUSTACHE

In addition to Hitler's polishing his oratorical and political skills, he also needed to make his personal appearance more distinctive. If he was to become the leader of a Greater Germany, he required a few characteristic attributes. After all he was only five feet eight inches tall, and his frail physical appearance was not overly imposing. Hitler needed some characteristic features to set him off in the minds of his fellow Germans. He determined that one of his aspects was to exhibit a distinctive mustache.

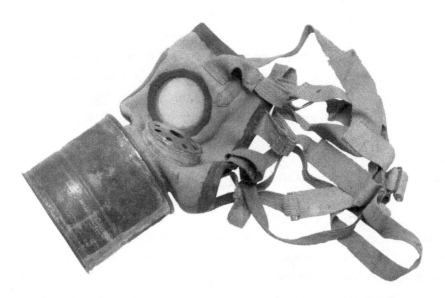

Illustration of typical German gas masks in World War I. (Alamy stock photo)

At the time he entered the German Army, Hitler sported a bushy, handlebar Kaiser mustache, styled after German emperor Kaiser Wilhelm II. Many German men wore this flamboyant, broad, and sometimes upturned-at-the-ends facial decoration. The extravagant nature of the mustache, however, made it difficult to maintain during wartime. For that reason, Hitler snipped off the ends of his Kaiser mustache and shaped it into his notorious toothbrush mustache.

An alternative but complementary explanation describes how Hitler during his service in World War I snipped off his Kaiser mustache to fit beneath his gas mask. This alteration would have reduced the risk of air leakage around the edges of the gas mask. Hitler's commander may have even ordered this adaptation over safety concerns for his troops given the contemporaneous introduction of gas attacks. Hitler's later injury in an English mustard gas attack bespoke the wisdom of such a directive.

The toothbrush mustache did not extend beyond the width of the nose and was well within the confines of the German World War I gas mask. Hitler shortened his mustache even more than was typical at the time to make himself more distinctive.

In later years he defended his more prominent modification by saying that this narrower mustache set him apart from the more typical toothbrush mustaches. Before Hitler's style of mustache became popular, in Bavaria it had often been called a *Rotzbremse* or snot brake.

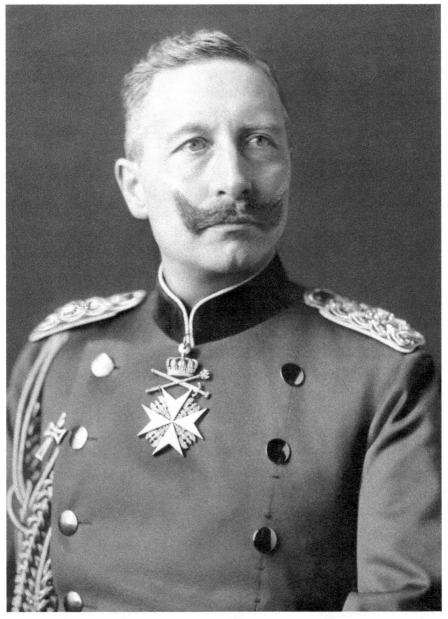

An example of the Kaiser mustache, popular prior to World War I but that would not fit under the gas mask. (Alamy stock photo; HU 68367 from the collections of the Imperial War Museums, www.wm.org.uk)

Hitler's abbreviated toothbrush mustache has also been referred to as a Charlie Chaplin mustache. Indeed, Charlie Chaplin wore his toothbrush mustache earlier than did Hitler, as he acquired his around 1915. Some have speculated that Hitler might have shaped his mustache after Chaplin, but this explanation seems doubtful. It is unlikely that Hitler would have adopted the likeness of a silent film comedian as such an imitation would have opened him up to ridicule. Being laughed at would have been antithetical to Adolf Hitler's great emotional need for respect.

THE EYES

A second physical characteristic that set Hitler apart was his eyes. Robert Waite in his 1976 book described Hitler's eyes as extraordinarily light blue in color with a faint touch of greenish gray. His strangely compelling eyes impressed almost everyone who met Hitler and were often commented upon. Hitler was aware of the impact that his eyes had on others and was known to practice piercing gazes by looking in the mirror. Women in particular became mesmerized, impressed, or frightened by Hitler's gaze. August Kubizek recalled:

> The eyes were so outstanding that one didn't notice anything else. Never in my life have I seen any other person whose appearance—how shall I put it—was so completely dominated by the eyes. They were the light eyes of his mother but her somewhat staring, penetrating gaze was even more marked in the son and had even more force and expressiveness. It was uncanny how those eyes could change their expression, especially when Adolf was speaking. In fact, Adolf spoke with his eyes, and even when his lips were silent one knew what he wanted to say. When he first came to our house, and I introduced him to my mother she said to me in the evening "What eyes your friend has!" And I remember quite distinctly that there was more fear than admiration in her words. If I am asked where one could perceive, in his youth this man's exceptional qualities, I can only answer, "In the eyes."

HITLER: THE RECRUITER

Despite being personally unpopular in the army and his prior failure as an artist, Hitler developed a remarkable capacity to recruit talented people. A few of his better-known colleagues whom he identified through the years will be discussed, providing insight into how Hitler chose his close associates.

During the political uprisings in Germany following World War I, Hitler came across a left-leaning political agitator by the name of Joseph Goebbels. After having

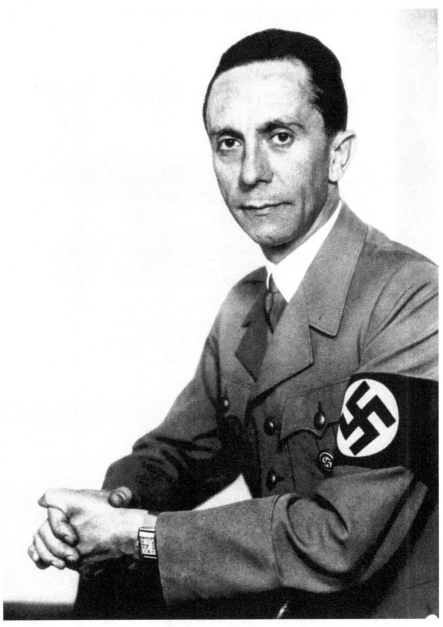

Portrait of Joseph Goebbels in his Nazi uniform. Goebbels was Reich Minister for Public Enlightenment and Propaganda, Gauleiter Berlin, Germany. (Alamy stock photo; Bundesarchiv, Bild 183-1989-0821-502 CC-BY-SA 3.0)

come under the persuasive influence of Hitler, Goebbels would go on to become an intellectual pillar of the Nazi Party and its chief propagandist. His talent for propaganda is still recognized today and much copied. Sharyl Attkisson in her 2017 book *Smear* credits Goebbels with perfecting propaganda techniques that have stood the test of time.

Goebbels's techniques as listed in his diaries include:

"A lie told once remains a lie, but a lie told a thousand times becomes the truth."

"Not every item of news should be published. Rather must those who control news policies endeavor to make every item of news serve a certain purpose."

"The truth is the greatest enemy of the State."

"It is an absolute right of the State to supervise the formation of public opinion."

"Propaganda must facilitate the displacement of aggression by specifying the targets for hatred."

Goebbels's effective use of these techniques played a huge role in helping Hitler to mobilize a war-averse German nation. Hitler completely captured the loyalty of Goebbels, such that when in 1945 he was trapped in Berlin with his wife and six children, rather than even attempt escape, the ever loyal and fanatical Goebbels chose to kill his children with cyanide and then take his and his wife's lives. Such was Goebbels's unflinching devotion to the Nazi cause and to Adolf Hitler.

Hitler also recognized the talent of Hermann Göring. This German hero aviator of World War I certainly looked the part of the ideal Nazi soldier. He was tall, handsome, brave, and, much to Hitler's liking, obedient to Hitler's wishes. In fact, Göring was the only member of Hitler's inner circle who could have met the physical requirements that had been established to join the *Schutzstaffel* (SS). Only much later did this ostentatious Hitler sycophant fall victim to greed, corruption, gluttony, and opiate addiction.

Göring would eventually become Reich Marshal and Commander in Chief of the German Air Force (Luftwaffe) but would fail abysmally in his attempts to bomb England into submission. His lack of success, as we shall see in subsequent chapters, was a major stumbling block to Hitler's achieving victory in World War II.

In 1931 Hitler also identified Albert Speer as a great talent in architecture and eventually appointed him Reich Minister of Armaments and War Production for Nazi Germany. Speer was an early supporter of Hitler and later spent as much personal time during World War II with Hitler as anyone in Hitler's inner circle. In addition to being a respected architect and creating magnificent architectural plans for the Reich Chancellery, the Zeppenfeld stadium in Nuremberg where the

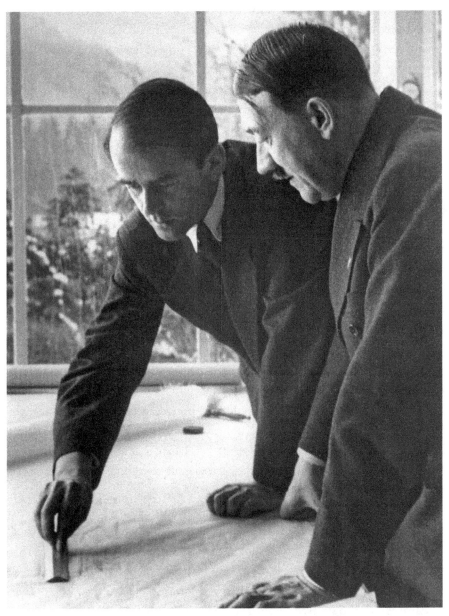

Albert Speer showing Hitler his design for the new Linz opera house. (Alamy stock photo; Bundesarchiv, Bild 183-2004-1103-500 / CC-BY-SA 3)

great Nazi rallies were held, and the reconstruction of Berlin and Linz on grand scales, Speer proved to be an amazingly efficient administrator. Despite nearly ceaseless bombing from the Allies, Speer, as Minister for Armaments and War Production, managed to keep the war materials flowing until very near the end of the war.

Speer was steadfastly loyal to Hitler. Only at the Nuremberg trials did he come to recognize or admit the immorality of the Nazi regime. For his crimes he served twenty years in Spandau prison, largely for the crime of having used forced labor during the war.

Adolf Hitler certainly had an eye for talent and an ability to recruit talented people who would loyally do his bidding.

PSYCHOLOGICAL EXPLANATIONS ON BECOMING HITLER

Several psychologists, psychoanalysts, and psychiatrists have offered insights as to how the youthful Hitler turned into the mature, depraved man that he eventually became. These opinions differ in some instances and cannot be altogether accepted. They approach the description of Hitler's personality from different aspects. Some of the psychoanalytic formulations seem rather fanciful and are hard to accept. Nevertheless, an in-depth look at Hitler's behavioral makeup from the various perspectives provides valuable information on interpreting the man.

It is at least of historical interest that, according to Morris Leikind's declassified report, the American intelligence community believed Hitler insane. It was felt that the outstanding characteristic of Hitler that dominated all others was that he was a man of violent passions. According to Leikind, Hitler's temper tantrums as a child, rather than going away as would be expected, instead evolved to become ever more virulent with his frenzies, his bitterness, and his animosities becoming legendary. Some historians lately have made the case that at least some of these tirades as an adult were more theater than actual pique, although many instances of Hitler's rage have been well documented.

Alice Miller, as previously mentioned, provided a better-reasoned and more advanced understanding of Hitler's behavior than did Leikind. She postulated the "humiliated child" theory. In short, Adolf's humiliation by his father and his father's withholding of love were thought to have brought about a brooding anger that later played itself out in Hitler's destructive ways.

Alice Miller also stressed that Klara's sister, who was schizophrenic and physically stooped, and who lived with the Hitler family, had a substantial detrimental influence on Adolf. Young Adolf disliked and feared her. This sister of Klara demonstrated bizarre behavior and terrorized Adolf. Her conduct by itself might have been better accepted had Adolf's parents been more emotionally present for him and explained the crazy aunt's comportment and, by so doing, allowed young Adolf to vent his emotional distress.

Miller quotes Franz Jetzinger, author of *Hitler's Youth*, who had interviewed Franziska Hürl, a servant in the Hitler household when Adolf was born. Jetzinger learned from Franziska Hürl that she had quit her job in the Hitler home simply because she could not put up with this deranged aunt any longer. Hürl stated that she refused to be around "that crazy hunchback."

Miller speculates on the impact that this irrational, deformed aunt had on the psyche of young Adolf. She ventures that his hated aunt played a role in Hitler's later development of the German euthanasia laws, where many institutionalized individuals with major deformities and mental conditions were put to death.

Nevertheless, eugenics was widespread throughout Europe and in the United States even before Hitler adopted it. Many persons at the time believed that the Great War had taken out the best men and that countries needed to adopt positive measures (eugenics) to correct this demographic imbalance. Thus, substantial societal support already existed for eugenics when Hitler adopted what he viewed as a scientific approach for improving society.

Helm Stierlin offered a slightly different interpretation of Adolf Hitler's psychological development. Stierlin was a psychiatrist with great interest in family dynamics. He believed family transactions were vital in shaping and misshaping the personalities of their offspring. He emphasized that Adolf's mother had a disturbed and deprived childhood and was pushed out of the family at an early age to become the housekeeper/mistress of her future harsh and neglectful husband, Alois. Stierlin argues that her perspective brought her initially to cater to her son, and later to bind him to her by delegating to Adolf the task of providing meaning for her mundane and commonplace life. Adolf may have become the "avenger" for his beloved mother's difficult life with her limited opportunities.

Alois Sr., Adolf's father, was born out of wedlock, arguably may have been half Jewish, and beat Adolf frequently—some sources claim on almost a daily basis. Hitler's father instilled bitterness and hatred in Adolf that Stierlin believes, given the possible Jewishness of Alois, may have spilled over into the monstrous depths of Adolf's anti-Semitism.

Robert Waite described Hitler as having a borderline personality, meaning that the person shows features in between neurosis and psychosis. He believed that while Hitler was mentally ill, he could still function in some areas and with great effectiveness. People with borderline personality characteristically show paranoid tendencies. They distrust and are highly suspicious of others and consider themselves to be especially privileged. Those with borderline personalities may fantasize about their magical omnipotence and believe they have the right to exploit others.

Waite describes a splitting of the ego in borderline personality such that they may demonstrate cruelty and kindness, sentimentality and hardness, creativity and destructiveness. They may swing violently between protestations of love and wild bursts of hatred.

Psychiatrist Fritz Redlich provided a psychopathological review of Hitler and his life. He believed that while the individual diagnoses of antisocial behavior, borderline disorder, narcissistic disorder, and hysterical disorder were inadequate, each carried an important aspect of Hitler's behavior. Redlich favored interpretations of Hitler as having been a destructive, paranoid but charismatic leader whose supporters proved fanatical and the population sufficiently gullible to accept his false myths. He provided a diagnosis of Hitler as a "destructive and paranoid prophet."

Leonard Heston, a neuropsychiatrist, along with Renate Heston delved less into psychiatric diagnosis and more into the role that medication, especially methamphetamine, played in Hitler's altered behavior. They avoided any single psychiatric diagnosis but emphasized various aspects of Hitler's personality including his morbid anger, impulsiveness, abnormal progression and content of Hitler's thinking, over-focus on detail, mental rigidity, disorganization, suspiciousness, mood disorder with prominent mood swings, and grandiosity. Examples of several of these personality characteristics have already been given and others will be described in future chapters along with Hitler's performance as *der Führer*.

These various psychological, psychoanalytical, and psychiatric interpretations are more complementary than exclusionary. These aspects of Hitler's personality provide an undergirding for Hitler's thoughts and behaviors, and in addition predicted how he would respond to his unfolding health issues. While these personality traits are essential in explaining Hitler's role in history, they in no way become excuses for his destructive choices. While Hitler had abnormal personality characteristics, they did not rise to the level of a psychosis with a loss of contact with reality and they fail to provide medical excuses for his evil ways.

Hitler's time in Munich crystallized his personality. The Nazi Party, like the army before it, had become a new emotional "home" for Adolf Hitler as his connection to his nuclear family had been lost. From Munich he advanced with his adult personality intact, with an undying love for the Nazi Party, and with his career direction firmly established.

CHAPTER 7

GENERAL HEALTH

U p until this point, I have dealt mainly with Hitler's behavioral development along with his family medical history and social history. We now transition to a consideration of Adolf Hitler's adult and general medical concerns.

PREMONITIONS OF AN EARLY DEATH

Early in life Adolf Hitler became convinced he would never live into old age. His belief likely stemmed from several sources. His mother only lived to the age of forty-seven, dying young from cancer. Also, when Adolf was only a year old, his younger brother Edmund died of measles. Indeed, four of his siblings died as children, most from infectious diseases. Perhaps it is not that surprising, given the amount of death that young Adolf witnessed, that he too assumed he would succumb to a premature death. His premonition helps to understand his over-concern with his minor illnesses.

Later in Hitler's life at least twenty-one assassination attempts were undertaken prior to the Col. Claus von Stauffenberg bomb plot of July 20, 1944. Google lists a total of thirty-two separate attempts to kill Hitler starting in 1921; however, the exact number is uncertain and varies from report to report. Some attempts were carried out with pistols and others with bombs. Hitler's SS performed incredibly well in frustrating these many, varied assassination attempts.

With each failed assassination attempt, the likelihood of an early death must again have crossed Hitler's mind. Recognizing the number of plots on his life, some of Hitler's "paranoia" seems justified.

INJURIES

Despite the amount of carnage associated with the assassination attempt on July 20, 1944, by Col. Claus von Stauffenberg and other disgruntled military officers,

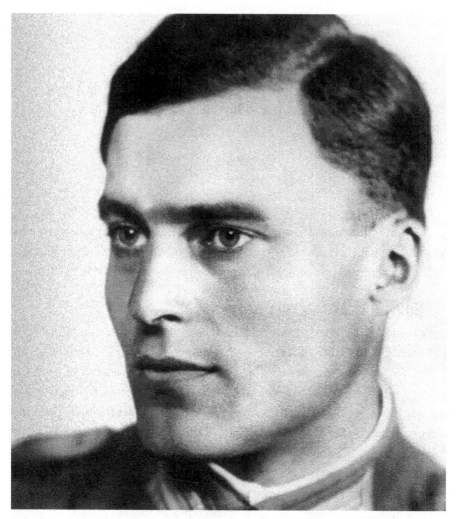

Col. Claus von Stauffenberg, who narrowly failed to assassinate Hitler on July 20, 1944. (Alamy stock photo)

Hitler received only relatively minor injuries. This was due to a massive oak table that largely protected him from the exploding bomb. The bomb had been hidden in a satchel that inadvertently had been kicked under the table next to a thick oak brace. The explosion left Hitler with many splinters in his legs along with bruises, abrasions, and bleeding from both ears due to perforated eardrums. Hitler lost the hearing in his right ear and ended up with diminished hearing in his left ear as well.

Hitler's narrow escape from this unsuccessful assassination attempt may have further convinced him that he was still destined to lead Germany to greater successes. His survival likely reinforced his belief that he lived a charmed, even messianic life. His continued existence was proof enough of the correctness of his supernatural experience from the military hospital at Pasewalk that had challenged him to become the savior of Germany.

JAUNDICE

In the autumn of 1944 while at Wolf's Lair (the code name for Hitler was Wolf) in eastern Prussia, he developed another medical problem—jaundice. Dr. Erwin Giesing (an ear, nose, and throat specialist), Dr. Karl Brandt (Hitler's general surgeon), and Dr. Hans Karl von Hasselbach (another assistant physician to Hitler) believed the jaundice resulted from the strychnine-containing (Dr. Koester's anti-gas) pills that Hitler routinely ingested for his chronic abdominal complaints.

Theodor Morell, Hitler's personal physician, was accused of prescribing the pills in question. At first Morell denied that the jaundice was even present, but when he could no longer ignore the obvious yellowish discoloration of Hitler's eyes and skin, the doctor began to argue vehemently against the jaundice having resulted from this medicine. He claimed the medicine was an over-the-counter preparation that he had not even prescribed but Hitler had obtained on his own. Instead, Morell maintained that an obstructed gall bladder had caused Hitler's jaundice.

Given the human crowding in the compound and uncertain sanitary conditions, hepatitis A also remains a possibility for Hitler's jaundice. Regardless of the correct diagnosis, Hitler had recovered fully from his jaundice by October 1944, and no further instances of jaundice occurred during his lifetime.

POSSIBLE HYPOSPADIAS

Recalling that Adolf's parents Alois and Klara were second cousins, the possibility of congenital malformations needs at least brief consideration. The offspring of second cousins slightly increases the risk of congenital malformations (from 2 to 3 percent up to around 5 percent). Whereas Adolf had no known visible malformations, speculation has existed regarding a possible hidden malformation, such as a penile abnormality (most likely hypospadias).

Hypospadias is the second most common congenital abnormality in the male reproductive system and consists of the urethral opening not being at the tip of the penis but rather underneath its tip. Hypospadias can make urination from a standing position difficult and can also lead to erectile dysfunction.

Hans-Joachim Neumann and Henrik Eberle in their book *Was Hitler Ill?* refer to the alleged hypospadias as myth, whereas Fritz Redlich favors its existence. If indeed Hitler had this congenital malformation, it would have caused urinary leakage and could possibly explain Hitler's habit of frequent hand washing. It could also explain Hitler's apparent limited interest in having sex, as with the abnormality he might have been impotent.

According to a study conducted by D. E. Sandberg and others (published as "Boys With Hypospadias: A Survey of Behavioral Difficulties" in 1989), boys from six to ten years of age in his study with hypospadias had more behavioral problems and lower social competency than those in a control group. More severe forms of hypospadias were associated with increased behavioral problems and still poorer school performance. While Adolf's poor school performance and behavioral outbursts are consistent with the behavior described with hypospadias, no documentation exists that Adolf had this congenital abnormality.

Throughout his life Adolf Hitler was excessively modest and might conceivably have prevented his doctors from examining his genitalia. As such, hypospadias remains a possibility. His seeming lack of interest in sexuality also might be explained by such a deformity due to either embarrassment or erectile dysfunction if it even existed. (Hitler's sexuality will be further discussed in chapter 9.)

CHRONIC ABDOMINAL COMPLAINTS

No medical problem gave rise to greater day-to-day distress and embarrassment for Adolf Hitler than did his lifelong abdominal disorder. This complaint increased in 1929, although he had similar, but less severe, problems as a child.

Following eating, Hitler would routinely develop abdominal pain, belching, a bloated sensation, and prominent flatulence. This complaint worsened in 1931 following the mysterious death of Hitler's niece, Geli Raubal, who some have claimed was the only woman, other than his mother, that Hitler truly loved.

It was following this stressful interlude after Geli's death that Hitler's bowel problems provoked him to become vegetarian. His abdominal complaints again increased in 1933, as Hitler maneuvered to improve his political position. This period of political maneuvering to become chancellor was a stressful period. Stress clearly played a role in the aggravation of his abdominal complaints, a fact not missed by his doctors who believed his bowel problems to be psychosomatic.

Hitler's symptoms are suggestive for what today is termed irritable bowel syndrome (IBS). While not life threatening or causing pathological changes in the intestinal tract, IBS is an uncomfortable condition and diminishes the quality of life. The cause of IBS is unknown. Often IBS symptoms can be controlled through dietary changes, lifestyle alterations, and stress reduction.

An amusing anecdote comes from *Uncle John's Endlessly Engrossing Bathroom Reader* by Miss Cellania that humorously described his attacks of flatulence. Hitler is described as periodically beating a hasty retreat from a room full of people and disappearing without explanation to privately pass bowel gas. The article claimed his flatulence was embarrassing and disturbing for both Hitler and those around him. His gassiness may have caused Hitler to swear off meat and to become a vegetarian. This change in diet failed to stop his flatulence but presumably made his bowel gas less malodorous. The article succumbed to the irresistible temptation of referring to Reich Chancellor Adolf Hitler as the richly alliterative "Fartin' *Führer*."

It is unclear if specific foods prompted his abdominal symptoms, but they may have followed consumption of fatty foods. If so, this would suggest gall bladder disease or irritable bowel syndrome. Unfortunately, Hitler did not allow diagnostic testing that might have secured a firmer diagnosis.

As mentioned earlier, his episodes of the most severe abdominal complaints roughly mirrored stressful episodes in Hitler's life. For this reason, Morell and other attending doctors assumed the symptoms were psychosomatic in origin. Morell essentially diagnosed chronic irritable bowel syndrome, and this diagnosis by today's medical standards seems reasonable.

Morell began treating Hitler with spasmolytics (medicines that relieve the intestinal spasms) and analgesics (pain relievers). Unfortunately for Hitler, the analgesics were largely opioids, causing the intestinal tract to reduce its motility, further aggravating Hitler's constipation and leading to still greater flatulence.

Following an evaluation of a sample of Hitler's stool, Morell began treatment with Mutaflor (the materialistic Morell was part owner of the company that made this worthless drug). This emulsion of a particular strain of bacteria taken from the feces of healthy Bulgarian peasants was meant to recolonize Hitler's GI tract with health-providing organisms. Despite the off-putting nature of the medicine's origin, it held a strong appeal for Hitler. Subsequent work on Mutaflor has determined that the medicine provided no benefit.

Morell, the always-enthusiastic prescriber of medicines, also used a mixture of laxatives and opioids to alternatively whip into action and then to rein in the movement of Hitler's bowels. This constant urging on and slowing up of the normal intestinal motility contributed to Hitler's GI problems and further aggravated his ongoing discomfort.

Belladonna was an ingredient in Dr. Koester's anti-gas pills and reduces the motility of the overactive bowel. In retrospect most experts favor the diagnosis of IBS and believe Morell was correct in his understanding of Hitler's abdominal disorder, if not his overall treatment of it.

CHAPTER 8

DID HITLER HAVE JEWISH BLOOD?

itler wrote in *Mein Kampf* that Jews were responsible for spreading syphilis. He disseminated this misinformation widely and simultaneously damned the Jews. Early in the twentieth century the cause of syphilis was determined to be an infectious agent, *Treponema pallidum*. Hitler, never known to be an extensive reader, may have remained unaware of this scientific discovery. Nevertheless, he continued a long tradition of using syphilis as slanderous propaganda.

The syphilis scourge had for centuries been attributed to a country's enemies. Syphilis became known as the "Spanish disease" by the Dutch, the "Italian disease" by the French, the "French disease" by the English, the "Polish disease" by the Russians, and the "Christian disease" by the Turks. In Hitler's instance, rather than damning an entire nation for the spread of syphilis, he chose his favorite target—the Jews.

An inordinate number of pages in *Mein Kampf* are devoted to the bane of syphilis. Much speculation has existed as to why Hitler held such an obsession and why he spent such an inordinate amount of time speaking and writing about it. Because of Hitler's clear obsession with syphilis and its association with Jews, an entire chapter will be devoted to this potentially insightful topic.

THE CASE FOR ADOLF HITLER HAVING A JEWISH GRANDFATHER

Whether Adolf Hitler had Jewish ancestors has great potential significance for understanding his actions. Alice Miller makes a convincing case for Alois Sr. having been the illegitimate son of Maria Anna Schickelgruber and a Jewish man from Graz, who possibly was named Frankenberger or perhaps Frankenreithner.

The man from Graz was wealthy and provided Maria Anna a regular monetary supplement. His stipend for her suggests either paternal support for Alois or hush money. The alleged Jewish father (or his son) likely did not wish to face public embarrassment by going to court and having to admit openly his sexual dalliance and out-of-wedlock offspring.

The money the wealthy man from Graz paid Maria Anna helped to financially support the poverty-stricken household in which Alois Sr. grew up. If Alois's father was Jewish, this knowledge or suspicion of it by Adolf could provide a basis for his anti-Semitism, as he loathed his father. Moreover, the culturally acceptable anti-Semitism of the time would have provided Hitler a ready excuse to justify the hatred he felt for his abusive father. According to some psychological interpretations, Hitler's initial dislike for his father may then have been transferred wholesale to the entire Jewish population.

PREVAILING ANTI-SEMITISM

In the Austria of Hitler's upbringing and in Germany at that time, it was common to hold anti-Semitic views. European governments and Christian denominations had for thousands of years sanctioned hatred of the Jews. The Jews also represented easy targets for repressed hate and unfulfilled aspirations.

Anti-Semitism was also a useful and effective political weapon that was widespread across much of Europe. This prejudiced mindset proved especially common following Germany's defeat in World War I when the Jews once again became prominent targets for scapegoating and were blamed for losing the war. Their crime according to the anti-Semitic bias lay in their involvement in banking and finance that ostensibly forced a premature cessation of the war.

Even during the Spanish Inquisition, Jews had been given the choice of accepting Christianity or facing torture and death. However, upon achieving ultimate power, Adolf Hitler gave no such leniency for religious conversion, deciding instead to remove any citizen rights from Jews, expel them, and later exterminate any who were still left in Greater Germany.

ADOLF'S ILLEGITIMATE FATHER

Hitler knew little for certain about his lineage. Considering the mores of the time, such things as illegitimacy were likely not openly discussed within the Hitler family and certainly not in front of the children. Acknowledgement of a Jewish ancestor and his father's out-of-wedlock birth would have been unthinkable topics for discussion with the proud Alois Sr. parked at the head of the dinner table.

Since Alois's mother was named Schickelgruber, the question arises as to why Alois was not called by his family name. Fritz Redlich, who has delved into this part of the family history, related the following:

> When Anna Maria Schickelgruber gave birth to Alois out of wedlock, she did not list the father's name at the time of the child's baptism or at any later time. Not long after giving birth, she moved into her parents' home. About five years later she married a mill worker, Johann Georg Hiedler. After Anna Maria's death, Alois lived with his prosperous uncle Johann Nepomuk Hiedler. Nineteen years later, Johann Nepomuk Hiedler asked the village priest to change Alois Schickelgruber's last name on his certificate of baptism to Alois Hitler, and further asked that Johann Georg Hiedler (his brother) be recognized as the father. He took three witnesses. One testified that Johann Georg Hiedler was Alois's father.

The delayed procedure in retrospect appears suspicious, and it was highly unusual at the time. Nevertheless, the church and state accepted the document with the three X's as signed by Johann Georg Hiedler, and Alois Schickelgruber officially became Alois Hitler.

Why the spelling changed for the similarly pronounced names, Hiedler and Hitler, is not entirely clear. It may have resulted from variable spellings of names in those days, a clerical error, a desire for literary economy, or due to different phonetic transcriptions. In any event Alois's offspring, Adolf Hitler, would become the most reviled name in the twentieth century.

Robert Waite also weighed in on whether Alois Hitler Sr. was half Jewish. In 1930 Adolf Hitler called in his personal lawyer, Hans Frank, to investigate his family history as Hitler was being threatened with blackmail by a relative. The relative claimed to have information to support the contention that Hitler had a Jewish grandfather. According to Waite, Frank discovered that indeed Hitler's father was illegitimate and that from Alois's birth until age fourteen, the Jewish family by the name of Frankenberger paid money for support of the child. No documents have been forthcoming nor have investigations occurred into whether any Frankenbergers even lived in Graz. Most historians studying this subject have concluded that we may never know for certain whether Hitler had Jewish blood.

Is there any wonder with such a confused family history that Adolf harbored suspicions throughout his life about who his real grandfather was, and whether he also had Jewish blood? Indeed, Hans Frank gave conflicting reports over his lifetime on the topic of Hitler's grandfather. Hitler also ordered an investigation by the race office of the *Schutzstaffel* (SS). The SS, to no great surprise, found *der Führer*, Adolf Hitler, to be one hundred percent Aryan. The validity of such a politically tinged report remains open to question.

POTENTIAL IMPACT OF HITLER'S HAVING JEWISH BLOOD

Alice Miller, who made the strongest case for Alois Hitler having been half Jewish, believed that Adolf transferred his repressed hatred for his father to the entire Jewish people. She believed this transference largely explains Hitler's shrill anti-Semitism.

On the other hand, Redlich could not confirm that Alois Sr.'s father was Jewish but also failed to confirm anyone else as his father. He believed Alois likely had a harsh upbringing and had been stubborn and doctrinaire. Alois Sr. also married three times, begetting eight children in wedlock and one illegitimate child.

Redlich described Adolf Hitler's obsession with the question of a "Jewish grandfather." Adolf Hitler took a remarkably personal interest in enacting the Nuremberg Law that prevented an Aryan woman younger than forty-five years of age from working in a Jewish household. This was the very situation in which his grandmother had found herself within the household of a Jewish man named Frankenberger or Frankenreithner. The rumor had it that either the father or son had impregnated her.

Whether or not Adolf Hitler had a Jewish grandfather remains unclear. What is clear is that Hitler recognized this eventuality as a very real possibility. His suspicion, rather than any certainty over his true family tree, drove his actions. Ample evidence exists that Adolf Hitler recognized the possibility of a Jewish grandfather, and via the psychological mechanism of transference, might have cruelly and catastrophically acted on his repressed suspicions.

Following the investigations into his ancestry later in life with the SS and his private attorney, Adolf Hitler declared he had absolutely no further interest in his family's genealogy. He proclaimed that he belonged to no one family but rather to the entire German nation. In effect, Hitler buried this question to avoid further speculation in Nazi-controlled Germany or elsewhere.

CHAPTER 9

HITLER'S SEXUALITY

W hile sexuality is not a physical or mental disorder, it is a significant enough aspect of a person's social history to include. The stigma attached to homosexuality during Hitler's time and homosexuality's perceived relationship to venereal diseases also makes this topic important for inclusion in this volume.

It has been variously asserted that Hitler had a normal sex life, was homosexual, and had sexual perversions. According to Robert Waite one major contribution that psychoanalysis has provided to historical biography is that sexual attitudes and practices play an important and integral part in personality development, and they shape a person's social thinking.

While we may never know for sure the details of Hitler's sex life, the importance of this aspect of his life for understanding the man warrants further coverage.

WAS HITLER HOMOSEXUAL?

Some writers have claimed that Adolf Hitler was gay. Given the intolerance of the times for homosexuality such an accusation, if broadly believed, would have constituted a fatal blow for Hitler's political career. If this claim was known to be true, Adolf Hitler would have kept it secret, as he was known to zealously protect his reputation.

It is helpful to review what is known and what is speculated regarding Hitler's sexual orientation. If Hitler was strictly homosexual, it would have diminished his likelihood of having contracted syphilis in 1908 from a female Jewish prostitute, as has been rumored. To be sure, Hitler's supposed infection by a Jewish prostitute has been magnified by rampant speculation and with little corroboration. Nevertheless, if valid, such an emotional cataclysm of contracting "the Jewish disease" predictably could have stoked Hitler's hatred and genocidal anti-Semitism.

While Germany tolerated homosexuality at times, it was historically viewed as a crime. Nowhere in German history was it dealt with as severely as it was during the Third Reich. Homosexuals, gay men more so than lesbians, were seen as sexual deviants and along with other "undesirables" rounded up, imprisoned, and sent to concentration camps. Conviction under the most stringent of the laws could even lead to castration. In the design to build the Aryan master race, homosexuality was seen as an obstacle in need of removal. Hitler referred to homosexuals as "disgusting creatures" and the laws imposed on homosexuals during the Third Reich were severe.

Despite the strong position against homosexuality by the Nazis, Hans-Joachim Neumann and Henrik Eberle argue that the overt display of virility under Nazism can be viewed as a homoerotic mass movement that included both men and women. The Nazis produced many morale-boosting videos of young, shirtless, handsome German men in shorts stretching and performing calisthenics and carrying out athletic endeavors. These videos, as well as demonstrating healthy and active young men, can be viewed as homoerotic. Neumann and Eberle suggest these are sexually charged videos that helped Hitler attract many gay men such as Ernst Röhm, an early leader of the *Sturmabteilung* (Stormtroopers, SA), to his service and proved politically useful for building up the movement.

Neumann and Eberle also hypothesize that the SS black uniforms, leather boots, leather belts and shoulder straps, and jack-booted troops with quirts in hand also smack of sadomasochism. Their harsh language and actions, abhorrence of undesirables, and overt cruelty were designed to convince both themselves and their onlookers that they represented an immutable force and a master race. To qualify for the SS, all recruits were required to be at least six feet tall, have blue eyes and light colored hair, and possess the appropriate Aryan facial features.

According to Waite, Ernst Röhm, the head of Hitler's Stormtroopers and a close friend of Hitler, was gay as was Rudolf Hess. Even though Hitler did not approve of homosexuality, he was a shrewd enough politician to understand that achieving his political goals trumped his antipathy to an important political assistant's personal behavior. In this instance Adolf Hitler was a political pragmatist, more so than a social zealot.

While Hitler eventually had Röhm killed, it was not for his sexual orientation but rather because Röhm had evolved into a potential political rival. Nevertheless, speculation has held that Röhm was able to blackmail Hitler due to Hitler's alleged homosexuality. This perceived threat is presumed to have led to Röhm's assassination in 1934 during the "Night of the Long Knives," an event in which

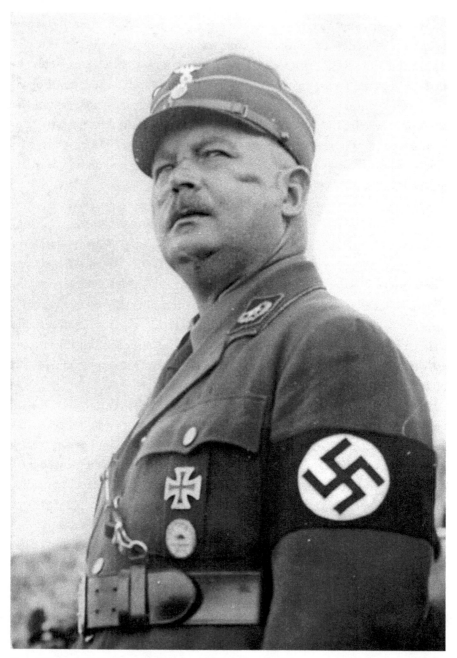

Ernst Röhm who, after having been one of Hitler's closest allies, was assassinated during the "Night of the Long Knives." His killing had more to do with his potential threat as a political rival than for his homosexuality. (Alamy stock photo; Bundesarchiv, Bild 102-15282A / Georg Pahl / CC-BY-SA 3.0)

Röhm—along with eighty-five others who represented either potential political rivals or witnesses to embarrassing episodes in Hitler's past—was assassinated.

Hitler biographer Lothar Machtan, along with Neumann and Eberle and others, described a supposed witness to Hitler's homosexuality. This narrative is the slenderest reed upon which to base Hitler's alleged sexual orientation. The informant, a man named Mend, was said to have billeted with Hitler in Flanders during World War I. He, like Hitler, was a dispatch runner. While staying at the Lefebvre brewery at Fournes, Mend claimed Hitler was caught during a homosexual encounter. When a light was unexpectedly turned on in the barn, Hitler and Schmidl (Ernst Schmidt) were found having sex in the hay. Mend scorned at the time, "Take a look at those two 'Nancy boys,'" an old euphemism for homosexuality.

Mend's veracity is open to question. As an aside, the term "Nancy boys" is believed to have derived from a burlesque comedian who pranced about the stage, acting as if he were gay. The character was a 1930s performer, after the time when Hitler was ostensibly found rolling in the hay. Mend's trustworthiness was discredited by his own later incarceration for sex crimes against women and children and his general lack of integrity. Following the war, Mend had considerable trouble with the law that included convictions for forgery and theft, and he eventually died in a German jail. Largely unsubstantiated rumors existed of Mend planning an extortion attempt by "outing" Hitler. As the conspiracy theory goes, this plot landed him in a German jail where he died under unknown but treacherous circumstances.

One thing about which nearly all writers concur was Hitler's low libido. Some historians have asked whether this characteristic might have resulted from his suppressed homosexual tendencies. Speculation has it that if he were gay, his relatively limited erotic interest in women would not be at all surprising. Providing some support for his limited interest in women and matters sexual were his comrades in World War I. Reports from them routinely attested to his indifference and prudery when speaking about sexual matters. Hitler was even referred to as a "monk." Hitler also had a striking dislike for sexual jokes and let his displeasure be known among his fellow infantrymen and later among his governmental and military underlings.

Later when Hitler became chancellor of Germany, his power and prestige attracted many women. He, like modern rock stars or movie stars, received large amounts of fan mail and love letters from adoring women that he could easily have converted into sexual trysts. The writers of some of these overt letters even offered to bear his child. He repeatedly ignored these offers of sex. Whether his rejections resulted from a lack of sexual drive, prudery, or fear of damage to his reputation is unknown.

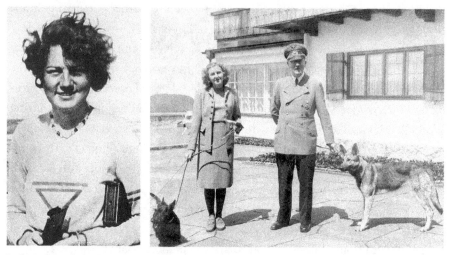

Left: Geli Raubal, who may have been, other than his mother, the only woman Hitler truly loved. (Alamy stock photo; LC-USZ62-74837) Right: Eva Braun and Adolf walking their dogs. (Alamy stock photo; Bundesarchiv, B 145 Bild-F051673-0059 / CC-BY-SA)

WAS HITLER HETEROSEXUAL?

Stronger support exists for Hitler being heterosexual than do rumors for his homosexuality. Hitler is believed to have had sexual relationships with multiple women including his niece Geli Raubal, Magda Goebbels (wife of Germany's Propaganda Minister Joseph Goebbels), Leni Riefenstahl, Winifred Wagner, a film actress named Renate Berchtesgaden, Lady Valkyrie Mitford (an English socialite and Nazi supporter who became part of Hitler's inner circle), Inge Ley (wife of Robert Ley, a prominent and unswervingly loyal Nazi politician and head of the German labor movement), Susi Liptauer, Martha Dodd (daughter of the US ambassador to Germany), and Maria Reiter. Maria Reiter—commonly called "Mimi" or "Mitzi"—claimed she was only a sixteen-year-old shop girl in Obersalzberg when she first met Hitler, who at the time was thirty-seven years old. She was the only woman who documented a reasonably clear description of sexual relations with Hitler.

Hitler had tried at the time to press Mimi into becoming his mistress, but she demurred. After she later separated from her husband, Reiter and Hitler reestablished a personal relationship. She described a sexual episode with Hitler as follows:

> He pressed me to his body and kissed me. It was well past midnight. He leaned back more and more on his sofa. Wolf (Hitler's nickname) grabbed me even more firmly. I let anything happen with me. I was never as happy as during that night.

All contacts with these other women preceded his relationship with the long-suffering Eva Braun. She hinted broadly, using modest and obscure diary references, to a sexual relationship with Hitler.

When loitering outside the bedroom occupied by Hitler and Eva Braun, Rochus Misch, who was Hitler's bodyguard, recalled hearing unmistakable orgasmic sounds. This audible clue suggests Hitler enjoyed a sexual relationship with Braun.

More so than explicit sex, the most remarkable feature of Hitler's relationship with women is the number of violent deaths that occurred with the women. Geli Raubal, Hitler's niece and mistress whom he had put up in a Munich apartment, died of either a self-inflicted gunshot to her chest or possibly a Hitler-caused homicide. This event almost derailed Hitler's budding political career at the time. Later Charles Trueheart, reporting on Ron Rosenbaum's book *Explaining Hitler* (1998), resurrected the story in a *Washington Post* article.

After the girl was found dead in her bedroom in Adolf's apartment in Munich on September 19, 1931, Hitler's staff conducted a clumsy cover-up. Only a limited autopsy was performed. Whether Geli's death was truly suicide, as it was officially listed, or a murder, we shall likely never know. Allegations existed that Geli might have been pregnant by a Jew, setting off a homicidal rage in Hitler.

In addition to Geli's death, Eva Braun, Lady Valkyrie Mitford, Susi Liptauer, and Maria Reiter all attempted or were successful at committing suicide. By any measure these women represent an extraordinary number of suicides, suggesting personal despair after having a sexual relationship with Adolf Hitler. These suicides have naturally prompted speculation about Hitler's inability to provide love, emotional intimacy, and nurturing for the women in his life.

Hitler's private physician, Theodor Morell, thought Hitler was sexually potent. According to Hitler's private medical record, Morell prescribed testosterone preparations of his own making to enhance Hitler's virility. Who instigated such treatment remains unclear. Did Morell carry out this treatment to increase Hitler's virility to make him more assertive in his performance as chancellor? Alternatively, did Hitler recognize his lack of libido and wish to have it enhanced? It is even possible that Eva Braun urged Morell to provide treatment because of her concern about Hitler's diffidence toward having sexual intercourse with her. This is another instance where we may never fully know the answer to questions relating to Hitler's sexuality.

Of course, Hitler's likely heterosexual behavior offered a greater likelihood for catching a venereal disease from a female prostitute. Whether or not this ever occurred will be a topic of the next chapter.

WAS HITLER SEXUALLY POTENT?

Regardless of Hitler's sexual orientation, the question arises as to whether Hitler was even sexually potent. (Later in this book his major illnesses associated with lack of sexual potency are more fully explored.) Parkinson's disease has been shown, especially in the advanced stages, to have autonomic nervous system abnormalities that often cause impotence. Hitler also had vascular disease. Vascular disease is the principal cause of erectile dysfunction. Adolf Hitler suffered from high blood pressure that gives rise to atherosclerosis and stiffening of the arteries with blockage, leading to erectile dysfunction.

Many blood pressure medicines are known to have negative impacts on sexual function, but the medical record fails to reveal that Hitler was treated with any medicines containing this side effect. Treatment for high blood pressure did not begin in earnest until the 1950s. The absence of treatment by Morell for high blood pressure can be viewed as standard medical practice for the day.

We may never know whether or not Hitler was troubled by impotence. This is certainly not something that the excessively private man would have openly shared with others. We do know that Morell prescribed for him a sexual tonic (Testoviron from Schering, a testosterone propionate in oil solution preparation). Morell injected this in 1943 and possibly 1944. This product was derived from pulverized bulls' testes.

Neumann and Eberle counted thirteen injections of Testoviron in May, four in September, and four in October 1943. This preparation was administered to Hitler, particularly when Eva Braun was around, suggesting a motive for this treatment. Hitler also received injections of Orchikrin and Prostakrin, both extracts of seminal vesicles and prostate of young bulls. Whether this triple therapy shows a heightened concern by Morell for Hitler's potency, or whether it is merely another example of Morell's enthusiasm for polypharmacy, believing if one medicine was good then multiple meds must be even better, is unknown. The latter two agents were from Morell's own pharmaceutical firm, also suggesting that Morell may have had a profit motive.

While these medicines might have boosted Hitler's energy and sense of wellbeing, the temporal relationship to the presence of his mistress is the strongest evidence suggesting Morell attempted to boost Hitler's sexual desire and performance.

HITLER'S ALLEGED SEXUAL HABITS

It is possible that Hitler's lack of apparent sexual desire for Eva Braun had more to do with his unusual sexual preferences than with Eva's sexual attraction per se.

Norbert Bromberg, a German-born psychiatrist and professor at Albert Einstein Medical School in New York, described in his book *Hitler's Psychopathology* (1987) the 1971 findings of Helm Stierlin, a prominent German psychiatrist, regarding the perverted sexual habits of Adolf Hitler as follows: "The only way in which he could get full sexual satisfaction was to watch a young woman as she squatted over his head and urinated or defecated in his face." Bromberg reported an episode in which Hitler became quite sexually charged during a sexual liaison with a young German actress. He described it as follows:

> . . . at whose feet Hitler threw himself, asking her to kick him. When she demurred, he pleaded with her to comply with his wish, heaping accusations on himself and groveling at her feet in such an agonizing manner that she finally acceded. When she kicked him, he became excited, and as she continued to kick him at his urging, he became increasingly excited.

Bromberg described Adolf Hitler's unusual sexual preferences, but he has been criticized for lack of corroboration and excessive speculation. However, a discussion of Hitler's sexuality would be remiss if it did not include this unverified and shocking assertion.

Nevertheless, early in World War II, Bill Donovan and the American Office of Strategic Services (OSS) prepared disinformation on Adolf Hitler, describing this very sexual perversion that was intended to malign the German dictator. It seems likely Bromberg and others may have been taken in by this OSS propaganda or even by Hitler's domestic political opponents such as Otto Strasser who may have covertly seeded such misinformation.

Dietrich Orlow, a professor of history at Boston University, wrote a book review in 1979 of *The Psychopathic God* by Robert G. L. Waite. In this review, Orlow took to task Waite's claim that Hitler was born with only one testicle that in turn gave rise to supposed fears of sexual inadequacy and incomplete manhood. This anatomical abnormality, along with reportedly having witnessed his parents having sex, drew heavily upon Freudian interpretation and gave rise to Waite's belief that these issues caused Hitler's virulent anti-Semitism. As will be discussed further in chapter 22, the one testicle theory is likely a fabrication of Allied propaganda and bogus Soviet forensic pathology.

To summarize, the evidence relating to Hitler's sexual orientation is murky. According to most authors Hitler was most likely heterosexual or possibly bisexual. Signs exist that he was largely asexual throughout his life due to the possibility of suppressed homosexual tendencies, a possible deformation of his genitals, or simply that he possessed diminished libido. What seems clear is that he had interest in multiple women for either sexual or decorative purposes but displayed a low libido and largely avoided sexual entanglements. He likely lacked the emotional equipment to nurture a relationship with a woman and proved a most disappointing choice for a soul mate.

CHAPTER 10

DID HITLER HAVE SYPHILIS?

Syphilis is a major medical illness that has both cardiac and neurological implications. In middle age Hitler developed both heart disease and the neurological condition of Parkinson's disease. Both conditions will be discussed in detail in coming chapters. Despite extensive writings about Hitler's purported syphilis, the question arises as to whether he had ever contracted this infectious malady and whether it gave rise to his heart and brain disease. Certainly, syphilis can act as a medical masquerader and deserves some consideration. As noted earlier, syphilis has also been used for centuries to slander both individuals and enemy countries. Likewise, Allied propaganda during World War II claimed Hitler had syphilis. But did he?

SYPHILIS RUMORS

The question of whether Adolf Hitler contracted syphilis repeatedly surfaces in writings about his life, health, and development of anti-Semitism. Few disorders have been more difficult to confirm or refute than syphilis, but it is important to exclude this purported illness to discuss more likely diagnoses.

An individual's sexuality can be a very private matter. To make clarification of the syphilis rumors even more difficult, Hitler was both exceedingly modest and scrupulously protective of his reputation.

In 2003, Deborah Hayden published an interesting book, *Pox: Genius, Madness, and the Mysteries of Syphilis*. This book contains a chapter on Adolf Hitler in which she builds a case for Hitler having developed an advanced case of syphilis that is known as general paresis. The author of this work is a talented writer and historian, but Hayden is not a physician. She dug into old, turgid treatises, and by using circumstantial evidence argues her case for Hitler having general paresis.

Hayden's book represents an ambitious attempt, as she states it, "to assemble the clues into a recognizable, repeatable pattern that would open the question [presence of syphilis] to debate." She posits that Hitler suffered from syphilitic general paresis (an old term indicating generalized weakness usually associated with insanity) such that it may have affected his performance as Reich Chancellor.

Hayden makes some good points, but retrospective diagnosis and the lack of serological proof, tissue samples, or appropriate neurological signs present huge challenges to her confirming this presumptive diagnosis. Hayden's indirect case for syphilis is nicely presented and, as she said, deserves further debate.

Syphilis is a sexually transmitted disease caused by a microorganism known as a spirochete. Syphilis is known medically as the "great imitator" and, as such, is often open to misdiagnosis. Syphilis may present with rashes, abdominal pains, muscular aches, neurological symptoms, heart symptoms, and even sores in the mouth. It is called the "great imitator" because it presents in many ways that suggest other diseases. The multiple stages of syphilis also differ in symptomatology from each other. With the possible exceptions of Ebola, the bubonic plaque, and leprosy, syphilis has given rise to more fear and misunderstanding than has any other medical disorder.

This chapter will briefly review what is known, or at least speculated, about Hitler's possible syphilis, including manifestations suggestive for neurosyphilis (the modern term for general paresis of the insane). In what follows we will determine in greater detail how these known characteristics of neurosyphilis match with Hitler's complaints and his findings on physical examination.

HISTORICAL CLAIMS

In *Inside the Third Reich* (1970), Albert Speer wrote that Hitler believed he had a powerful sexual appeal to women. Nevertheless, Hitler felt insecure about his appeal, not knowing if it rose from being the powerful chancellor of Germany or from his personal magnetism. In any event, it is not generally believed that he pursued the many potential sexual liaisons that he was offered, thus reducing opportunities for contracting the illness.

As also stated earlier, Hitler's low libido prompted hearsay regarding his sexual orientation that has an impact on his likelihood of contracting syphilis. Fevered propaganda during World War II by the Allies makes the subject of his sexual practices still more opaque and adds further difficulty for extracting truth from propaganda.

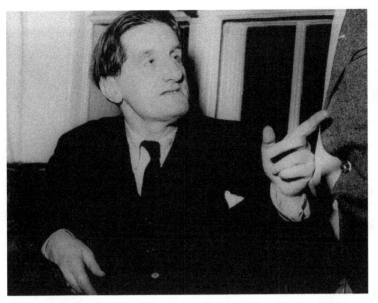

Ernst "Putzi" Hanfstaengl, Hitler's Harvard-educated foreign press secretary, who related stories of Hitler's possible syphilis. (Alamy stock photo; Bundesarchiv, Bild 183-R41953 / CC-BY-SA 3.0, CC BY-SA 3.0)

The rumors began with Putzi Hanfstaengl, a Harvard-educated friend of Hitler, who for years served as Hitler's foreign press secretary. In his memoirs, Hanfstaengl said that in 1908 a Viennese Jewish prostitute infected Hitler with syphilis. Moreover, Hanfstaengl claimed that Hitler had been infected because he didn't know enough not to ejaculate into the prostitute. Hanfstaengl clung to outmoded beliefs that the infective agent (a spirochete) could only enter a flaccid penis. Hanfstaengl was a clever, histrionic, and well-connected individual. It is difficult, lacking any real evidence and given his unreliable personality, to know how much credibility to attach to his gossipy claims.

Many years after the conclusion of World War II, a respected London expert in syphilis, Dr. T. Anwyl-Davies, conveyed a story that two men told him one night while the narrators were imbibing in a bar. The two men claimed the same prostitute who had infected Hitler had also infected them. The trustworthiness of this report remains in question. Nevertheless, Anwyl-Davies concluded that by the end of World War II Hitler was in the tertiary (most advanced) stage of syphilis.

Another possible clue regarding the rumored syphilis in Hitler arises from Hitler himself. While imprisoned for treason in Landsberg prison following the failed Beer Hall Putsch, Hitler wrote thirteen pages in *Mein Kampf* on the terrible scourge of syphilis. His devotion of so much space to this medical topic in a

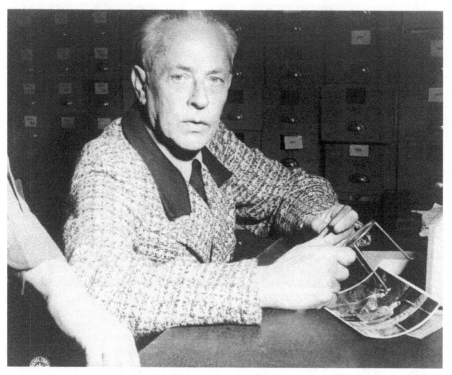

Heinrich Hoffmann, a friend of and photographer for Hitler, who developed gonorrhea. He brought to Hitler's circle the attractive young female assistant, Eva Braun. (Alamy stock photo; US Army Signal Corps, https://www.loc.gov/pictures/item/2005680418)

political screed, and his claim that syphilis was the direst threat facing humanity, has ever since caused a collective arching of the eyebrows. In *Mein Kampf*, Hitler stated: ". . . it must be considered that we often have to deal with visitors from the provinces who are completely befuddled by all the magic of the city." In this passage was Hitler referring to himself as being such a country bumpkin, fumbling and experimenting around in Vienna and as a result catching syphilis?

Hitler apparently believed syphilis was an inheritable Jewish disease. This notion was a common belief of the day. Did Adolf Hitler believe he might have inherited syphilis from his hated father who may have been half-Jewish? It has been speculated that Hitler felt the Jews had to be exterminated to rid the German nation of syphilis, a factually incorrect rationale but that arguably could have unleashed the Holocaust.

THE ROLE OF HEINRICH HOFFMANN'S VENEREAL DISEASE

In 1936, Hitler sent his personal airplane to Berlin on a singular mission of mercy. It was dispatched to procure Dr. Morell, a general physician, who although having no particular training in venereal diseases, was well known for treating venereal diseases among the rich, famous, and well connected. Heinrich Hoffmann, Hitler's friend and photographer, needed Morell's services for just such a sensitive situation.

Hoffmann had the misfortune to contract gonorrhea and, no doubt, was troubled by the typical symptoms of gonorrhea including discharge from his penis, frequency of urination, and pain. Hoffmann at the time was married to his second wife and had two children and must have harbored concerns about infecting his wife. He confided his embarrassing and discomforting condition to his friend, Adolf Hitler.

Shortly thereafter, Dr. Theodor Morell, who was to later become Hitler's self-serving private doctor, arrived at the Berghof—Hitler's residence in the Bavarian Alps—with medical bag in hand. There he provided treatments that cured a grateful Herr Hoffmann.

While visiting the Berghof, Morell became personally acquainted with Adolf Hitler and they developed a friendship. Both men had served in World War I and Morell was a member of the Nazi Party. No doubt, they had some common interests and likely swapped war stories. After a time, Hitler asked him to join his staff and become his personal physician.

Parenthetically, Hoffmann had an attractive, happy, young blonde female assistant who helped him in his work as a photographer. Her name was Eva Braun. Hitler took a liking to the carefree, nonpolitical, and reportedly empty-headed Eva, and Braun and Hitler went on to establish a romantic relationship. Her good looks, outgoing ways, and lack of interest in politics proved the polar opposite of Hitler's personality.

Hitler's choice of Morell as his personal physician has given rise to suspicion that Hitler might also have suffered from a venereal disease. Alternatively, Hitler may have simply liked Morell because he was medically unorthodox and willing to try novel, unverified treatments. To his advantage in Hitler's eyes, unlike many of the doctors in Germany Morell was not Jewish. Theodor Morell was, however, an avid social climber who saw Hitler as a fast track to wealth, success, and fame.

SYMPTOMS AND SIGNS OF POSSIBLE SYPHILIS

Hitler had many medical complaints. A short list of symptoms in his medical and historical records include headache, ringing of the ears, sinus problems, visual disturbances, hoarseness, belly pains, flatulence, skin rashes, tremor, high blood pressure, changes in his electrocardiograms, joint pains, emotional outbursts, and sleep difficulties. Syphilis can cause many symptoms including some listed. Given the breadth of Hitler's complaints, the "great imitator" syphilis could reasonably be considered a unifying diagnosis. Alternatively, Hitler may simply have suffered from what many of his doctors assumed were a variety of psychosomatic complaints or a collection of unrelated disorders.

Regarding a diagnosis of syphilis in Hitler, no clear medical reports exist to suggest it. Of great significance was that Hitler's case file contained a negative Wassermann test (as reported by David Irving in Morell's casebook).* This test was the prevalent serology used at that time to diagnose syphilis.

It can be argued that Hitler might have hidden an indiscretion from Morell but his Wassermann test, if positive, would have revealed its presence to Morell. Alternatively, if Morell had been made aware of a history of syphilis in Hitler, he conceivably might have guarded his need for privacy by not including the diagnosis even in Hitler's private medical record. Nevertheless, if Hitler chose Morell, a venereal disease doctor, because of his personal concerns with venereal disease, then it seems to reason that he would have mentioned his apprehension to his doctor.

Such are some of the potential mental machinations that describe the possible interaction of an extremely private patient and a secretive, socially upward driven doctor.

NEUROSYPHILIS (GENERAL PARESIS)

Deborah Hayden in her book suggested that Hitler had developed an advanced form of syphilis known as general paresis and that it impaired his performance as chancellor. This form of syphilis affects the brain and spinal cord and gives rise to a variety of symptoms including seizures, blindness, muscular weakness, tremor, emotional swings, psychoses, and dementia. Hitler had some of these symptoms, but closer inspection is required to determine if his physical findings confirmed a diagnosis of general paresis.

---

* David Irving for years enjoyed an excellent reputation as a respected World War II historian. He lost his good reputation over valid allegations that he had become a Holocaust denier and a historical revisionist. Indeed, he was involved in lawsuits that he lost that impoverished him. He even served a prison sentence in Austria.

In *The Secret Diaries of Hitler's Doctor*, Irving translated Morell's medical diary about patient Hitler and provided commentary on his illnesses. However, this work is believed by the current author to be scholarly in that it shows no evidence of Holocaust denial, praise of Hitler, or usage of misleading information. For that reason, this book of Irving's is used here as a reference to the role of Theodor Morell and with full knowledge of Irving's unsavory reputation.

Russell Brain and John N. Walton in *Brain's Diseases of the Nervous System* (1969) describe the medical problems that occur with this disorder. Seizures occur in 50 percent of cases. Muscular strength becomes progressively impaired. Tremor may be present in the outstretched extremities but is most conspicuous when the extremities are moving. Tremor typically affects facial muscles, lips, and tongue. Lack of coordination is usually seen in the advanced stages rendering the gait unsteady. Incoordination of the arms is also present but less evident to casual inspection. A progressive loss of body weight is expected. The optic nerves frequently degenerate and become pale on funduscopic examination (examining the back of the eye, the so-called optic discs, using an ophthalmoscope), giving rise to visual loss leading to blindness. While grandiosity (an unrealistic sense of superiority and disdainfully viewing others as inferior) is the best known of the mental changes, the dementing form is more common. A spinal fluid examination provides excellent diagnostic findings that, if present, are highly characteristic for syphilis.

DID HITLER'S SIGNS SUGGEST GENERAL PARESIS (NEUROSYPHILIS)?

How do Hitler's symptoms match up with the usual features of general paresis? Not well is the short answer. Nowhere in Hitler's medical records are seizures documented. The tremor he had involved his hands and was a slow, resting tremor, and not a tremor with action as is typical for general paresis. He did not show tremor of the facial muscles, tongue, or lips, which is the more common location of tremor with general paresis. No mention of muscle weakness of the sort seen with general paresis was documented, nor did he show incoordination of his arms or legs.

His gait was a shuffling type of gait and not an unstable (or ataxic) type seen with general paresis. The best-known gait abnormality of advanced syphilis is due to involvement of the back portion of the spinal cord responsible for sensing position of the limbs. This damage to the spinal cord gives rise to a characteristic slapping gait in which the forceful slapping down of the feet increases the sensation higher up in the legs to better sense leg position. Hitler did not demonstrate a slapping gait but instead showed a shuffling gait.

In addition, Hitler's medical records did not list optic atrophy (whiteness of the optic nerve due to degeneration) and he was examined repeatedly by ophthalmologists for his eye complaints. It is inconceivable that his ophthalmologists would have missed this obvious sign.

Hitler did not show a steady weight loss as expected with general paresis. He also had repeatedly negative Wassermann tests as well as negative Meinicke and Kahn tests (both syphilis serologic tests). He apparently never had an examination of his spinal fluid, a test that would have excluded the diagnosis, had the test been performed. Hitler also never showed dementia but may have had a milder Parkinson's related neuropsychological syndrome that will be described later and one that is characteristic for Parkinson's disease and not for syphilis.

The course of syphilis also may be helpful for differentiating Hitler's disorders from other illnesses. General paresis usually develops ten to fifteen years following infection by the microorganism and is rare to develop after twenty years. By 1941, when many of Hitler's neurological symptoms became evident, Adolf Hitler would have been thirty-three years out from his date of presumptive syphilitic infection. This latency is a much longer than would be expected for syphilis and strongly argues against syphilis as the cause of his neurological symptoms.

In summary, while syphilis can be a great imitator and deserves careful consideration, there exists too little evidence to suggest that Hitler suffered from syphilitic general paresis. The latency from presumed infection is too long, and the physical signs and laboratory tests fail to match up with the symptoms and signs in a fashion suggestive for general paresis.

Neurological diagnoses are made not only from symptoms but usually require confirmation by physical findings and laboratory corroboration. With a substantial degree of confidence, it can be said that Adolf Hitler did *not* suffer from general paresis (neurosyphilis).

No mention exists in Morell's case notes on patient Hitler about a diagnosis of syphilis or treatment thereof. A routine Wassermann test dated January 10, 1940, was negative, indicating an absence of syphilis. Likewise, Meinecke and Kahn tests, used to detect the presence of syphilis, were negative. These different types of negative tests represent convincing evidence that Hitler had never contracted syphilis.

Of course, Hitler may have thought he had contracted syphilis, given his tendency toward hypochondriasis. If indeed he held this conviction, then he might have developed an animosity against the Jewish prostitute and conceivably have generalized his hatred because of "the Jewish disease" to the entire Jewish population. It should be noted that during Hitler's time the belief existed that syphilis would affect ten generations of those who contracted the disease. Beliefs, true or false, still drive behavior. Is this why Hitler chose to not marry until immediately prior to his suicide given his concern over passing on bad traits to his offspring? It is likely we will never know his reasoning.

Finally, a note seems necessary on the rumored Jewish prostitute who ostensibly infected Hitler. It is overly simplistic to heap blame for Hitler's genocidal anti-Semitism onto a lone Jewish prostitute, if indeed she ever existed. Many other factors for his anti-Semitism may have been at work including the long-standing cultural anti-Jewish bias, the hated Jewish/Bolshevik movement as Hitler liked to allege, Adolf's antipathy toward the Viennese Academy of Fine Arts and its heavily Jewish faculty, and Hitler's perception of Jews as economic and cultural threats to the so-called Aryan people. These factors need to be weighed much more heavily than an unlikely diagnosis of syphilis when considering the origin of Adolf Hitler's anti-Semitism.

CHAPTER 11

HEART DISEASE

A side from minor general health concerns and the rumors of contracting syphilis, Adolf Hitler suffered from two major health problems: heart disease (discussed in this chapter) and Parkinson's disease (covered in later chapters). These two major illnesses affected not only his health but also his performance as the leader of Nazi Germany. These illnesses individually and in combination affected his expected length of life and his cognitive performance and may have impacted the eventual outcome of World War II.

As Adolf Hitler entered his fourth decade of life, he enjoyed good overall health. As mentioned earlier, his destructive personality had been firmly set during the 1920s but other than aches and pains resulting from his shrapnel wounds, his chronic abdominal complaints, and his periodic hoarseness, he remained vigorous and healthy during his thirties and early forties.

CORONARY SCLEROSIS AND HYPERTENSION

According to Theodor Morell's medical diaries, Hitler received a diagnosis of coronary sclerosis sometime prior to August 1941. This pathological condition begins with soft plaques forming in the coronary arteries of the heart and progresses to harder plaques that can block the flow of blood through the coronary vessels. These plaques also serve as a source for blood clots (emboli), leading to inflammation and heart attacks (myocardial infarctions). Today this condition is referred to as atherosclerosis of the coronary arteries or simply as coronary artery disease. It is a well-recognized cause for myocardial infarction and the leading cause of death in the developed world.

Professor Hans Karl von Hasselbach, a surgeon, joined Hitler's medical staff in 1936. Morell first examined Hitler on January 3, 1937. He made no mention of a blood pressure recording or heart sounds in that examination. According to

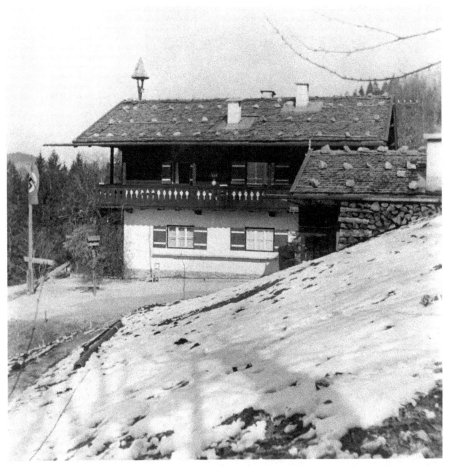

Picture of the Berghof in 1935, which lay high in the Bavarian Alps near Berchtesgaden, Bavaria, Germany. (Bundesarchiv, Bild 183-1999-0412-502)

David Irving's translations and commentary on Morell's medical diary, Hasselbach reported that Hitler had told him he had a weak heart.

Hitler was entering his late forties when Hasselbach joined the medical staff, and by this time Hitler had already learned to avoid climbing up to the Kehlsteinhaus high above the Berghof at six thousand feet in altitude. When Hitler had attempted this climb, he suffered a feeling of chest tightening. Hasselbach brushed off these symptoms as likely hysterical in nature, but it is certainly possible Hitler's sensation of chest tightening was the first clinical symptom of coronary artery disease, manifesting in what now is called exercise-induced angina pectoris. The combination of exercise that increases the demand for oxygenated blood and the thinning of oxygen at that elevation would aggravate symptoms of coronary artery disease.

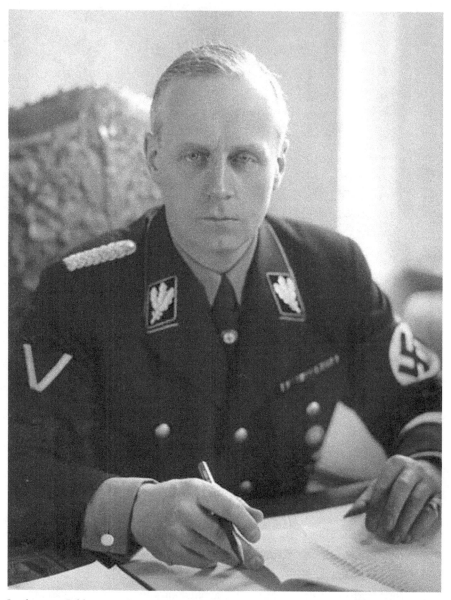

Joachim von Ribbentrop, German Foreign Minister. (Bundesarchiv, Bild 183-H04810)

Hitler's coronary disease was associated with elevated blood pressure (fluctuating moderate hypertension). Morell knew of the substantial risk of coronary artery disease for causing heart attacks and recorded it in his medical record as "a constant threat." Nevertheless, Morell minimized his risk assessment in Hitler's casebook by writing that it was not unusual in men his age. Morell's opinion seems unusual, as Adolf Hitler was only fifty-two when he assigned the diagnosis.

Hitler's coronary artery disease is known to have brought about clinical symptoms. In *Was Hitler Ill?* Hans-Joachim Neumann and Henrik Eberle describe a heated argument Hitler had with his foreign minister, Joachim von Ribbentrop, that occurred at the end of July 1941. This event led to Hitler suffering an attack of angina pectoris. These symptoms are identical to an impending heart attack and are associated with chest pain, shortness of breath, and pallor.

Apparently, Ribbentrop had summoned the audacity to question Hitler's wisdom in attacking the Soviet Union several months earlier, a country that possessed far greater resources in both men and warmaking abilities than did Germany. In addition, Ribbentrop had negotiated the Molotov-Ribbentrop Non-Aggression Pact of 1939 and felt personal qualms about breaking the treaty by attacking a former ally. Questioning the decision of a narcissist predictably brought forth an emotional outburst from Hitler.

Observers of the event described Hitler at first being thunderstruck by Ribbentrop's effrontery for having broached the impertinent topic, and then for having questioned the advisability of Hitler's decision. The color in Hitler's face drained such that he became pale. Hitler collapsed backward, falling into a chair while clutching his chest. After a short time, the color returned to Hitler's face.

"Don't ever again question any of my orders," Hitler said in a quiet voice, while recovering from the chest pain. He then continued, "I think I'm having a heart attack." This telling event provides convincing evidence for an attack of angina pectoris or possibly a mild myocardial infarction. At this juncture Hitler had not yet been prescribed nitroglycerin tablets but the attack subsided with time and rest.

Hitler had earlier informed Eva Braun, Albert Speer, and Joseph Goebbels that his heart was causing him increasing problems. He also reported his symptoms to Dr. Morell who ordered diagnostic studies. An electrocardiogram (ECG) was completed on Hitler on August 14, 1941 (the procedure was much harder to carry out then than it is now), and Morell arranged for it to be interpreted by the renowned cardiologist Dr. Arthur Weber on August 20 of the same year. Trying to maintain Hitler's privacy, Morell misled Weber by telling him that the unnamed patient was a diplomat from the Foreign Ministry. Weber interpreted the heart tracing as likely showing abnormalities of coronary sclerosis. Author Fritz Redlich, after gaining the opinion of cardiologist Richard Pasternak, wrote that this August 1941 tracing was also consistent with a small myocardial infarction.

Morell eventually ordered three other electrocardiograms performed on Adolf Hitler which were also interpreted by Weber. The second was performed in May 1943 and showed worsening of the myocardial repolarization abnormality. This

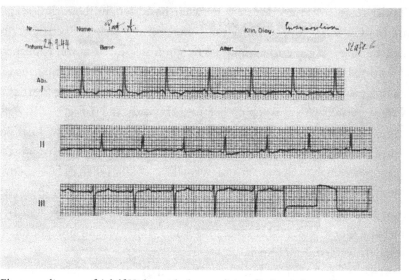

Electrocardiogram of Adolf Hitler, with abnormalities of ischemic heart disease, September 9, 1944.

electrocardiogram suggested an increase of the left ventricular hypertrophy (thickening of the walls of the left ventricle that pumps blood to the body) or myocardial ischemia (lack of blood flow to the heart muscle). The final two electrocardiograms in September 1944 were made using a "Master Step Test" in which Hitler stepped repeatedly on and off a two-step stool. This was the original cardiac stress test but only measured heart rate and the time it took the heart to recover following exercise. The test showed a degree of sophistication for its time.

Weber determined the series of ECGs suggested progressive worsening of the heart disease. Dr. Pasternak, as reported via Redlich, concluded that the cause of the ischemia was, likely, coronary heart disease (insufficient blood flow through the coronary arteries) in the presence of left ventricular hypertrophy—thickening of the left lower chamber of the heart that pumps blood to the body, as would be expected with long-standing high blood pressure.

In Weber's letter of May 17, 1943, he noted the deterioration in the ECG from the prior one. He advised the patient to rest for three or four weeks. If the patient was a smoker (Hitler did not smoke), he recommended this practice be discontinued. He also advised low salt in the patient's food and restriction of fluids. A further recommendation was for a regular afternoon rest and as much sleep at night as possible. These were standard recommendations in those days and could be given as well today. Nevertheless, today more modern diagnostic testing, intervention, and treatment would be offered.

At my request, Dr. James M. Wilson, a cardiologist at Baylor College of Medicine, in 2014 reinterpreted Hitler's electrocardiograms. Dr. Wilson interpreted the first one from 1941 as normal. While the diagnosis of "cardiac sclerosis" might in 1941 have been based on symptoms or physical findings, he found no evidence supporting it from the electrocardiogram.

The 1943 tracings differ from the one from 1941 with changes in the T-wave. According to Dr. Wilson a drug effect or an electrolyte abnormality are possible explanations but appear unconfirmed by the medical record. Worsening of Hitler's high blood pressure might also explain the change in the heart tracing. Real heart disease is also a possible explanation, but it is not provable by the initial 1943 tracing. Review of the medical record, however, supports the belief that the ECG changes resulted along with worsening heart disease.

According to Dr. Wilson, the 1944 tracing demonstrated more profound findings. The changes on this tracing were more specific for heart disease. The 1944 ECG and the serial studies argue strongly that Hitler had developed cardiac disease. Based on the ECG tracings, the possibilities include coronary artery disease, toxic myopathy (a disease of the heart muscle caused by a toxin), and hypertensive myopathy (enlargement and injury to the heart muscle due to long-standing high blood pressure).

Dr. Wilson argues that by the tracings alone we cannot ascertain a specific diagnosis of heart disease, but that progressive coronary artery disease is probable given the clinical information of Morell using nitroglycerin for the treatment of Hitler's symptoms. Nitroglycerin was used only for angina pectoris that was caused by coronary artery disease. Complaints of chest discomfort, difficulty breathing, and limitation of physical capacity as demonstrated by Hitler are confirmatory for a clinical diagnosis of coronary artery disease.

These restrictions served to remind Adolf Hitler that he was an ill man. Given the limited treatment available at the time, he must also have suspected and likely was told that his effective time to lead Germany was running out.

If Hasselbach's 1936 or 1937 estimation represents the onset of Hitler's symptoms of coronary artery disease, then the prediction of Hitler's expected survival would be in the range of 1944–1945. Hitler with his well-informed cadre of physicians could easily have ascertained his predicted shortened life stemming from his heart disease.

According to Ernst-Günther Schenck, a German physician and member of the SS in Nazi Germany who wrote a historically valuable memoir, nitroglycerin and digitalis were used to treat Hitler's heart disease. Schenck also summarized every injection and pill Morell gave Hitler from 1941 afterward. He reported, "Dr. Morell used 29 kinds of injections and 63 kinds of oral tablets and skin applications to treat Hitler."

The use went up dramatically after 1943 when the war in Russia began to turn against Germany. From Schenck and from review of Morell's medical diaries, Morell proved extremely enthusiastic in treating his demanding patient with a vast number of drugs. Morell at least tried everything known at the time to help with Hitler's heart disease. Nevertheless, Morell showed he was without concern for drug interactions or side effects.

SYPHILITIC DAMAGE TO THE AORTA

Deborah Hayden wrote that Hitler's symptoms relating to his heart disease most directly connected him to syphilis. She is correct that advanced syphilis may give rise to serious abnormalities of the heart and aorta since syphilis may cause ballooning of the first portion of the aorta (the large artery leaving the left ventricle of the heart) with occlusion or obstruction of coronary arteries, leading to shortness of breath and chest pain.

She appears incorrect, however, in her diagnosis of Hitler. With the advent of effective antibiotics, syphilitic aortitis (the medical diagnosis for this, referring to inflammation of the aorta due to the infectious agent) is now rarely encountered, but it was seen in Hitler's day. The widespread use of penicillin following World War II relegated syphilitic aortitis largely to the medical history books.

Hayden goes on to describe the reported abnormal second sound (aortic valve) that Morell mentioned in his medical notes of Adolf Hitler as being typical for inflammation of the aorta (syphilitic aortitis). Under interrogation after World War II, Morell stated he had heard via his stethoscope an "accentuation of the second aortic sound . . . in second intercostal space in the right parasternal line." Others have questioned whether Morell could discern such subtle changes in the heart sounds.

No record of a chest X-ray for Hitler exists. This is unfortunate for two reasons, as a simple chest X-ray examination would have determined if he ever had suffered from tuberculosis. It would also likely have been diagnostic for syphilitic aortitis by detecting a curvilinear calcium streak in the first portion of the aorta. Syphilitic aortitis gives rise to a ballooning of this portion of the aorta (aortic aneurysm). Today such an aneurysm would likely be resected, the incompetent aortic valve replaced, and coronary artery bypasses carried out, if needed, to address myocardial ischemia. Such procedures were of course unavailable during the 1940s.

Nevertheless, the blood pressure recordings for Adolf Hitler do not suggest aortic valve insufficiency (AI). With AI the systolic pressure is high, which contrasts with an abnormally low diastolic blood pressure. The low diastolic pressure is caused by blood flowing back through the incompetent aortic valve, thus reducing the pressure downstream. Dr. James Wilson concluded, based upon the absence of typical electrocardiogram findings associated with chronic aortic valve insufficiency, that he could reasonably exclude syphilitic aortitis with resulting aortic insufficiency.

While circumstantial evidence may suggest syphilitic aortitis, again a lack of medical evidence exists to adequately support a diagnosis of syphilitic heart disease in Adolf Hitler. Hayden's belief that Hitler's heart disease was due to syphilis, upon closer inspection, goes unsupported.

PROGNOSIS

As noted earlier, heart disease—whether it stemmed from the more likely atherosclerosis of the coronary arteries or from syphilitic heart disease—would have reduced Hitler's life expectancy. Symptomatic treatment with nitroglycerin would alleviate the chest pain that came on with exertion (angina pectoris). The description of Hitler's behavior at the time of the Ribbentrop argument proves strongly suggestive for a bout of angina pectoris due to coronary artery disease.

It is clear from Hitler's comments to others that he was greatly concerned about his heart and fretted about not living long enough to see his many plans enacted for achieving *Lebensraum*. Heart disease of this degree would have limited Hitler's physical activities as well as hasten his death.

Hitler's expectations and fear of a premature death were exacerbated by his awareness of his heart disease. Such knowledge would have created in him a sense of urgency for converting his messianic plan for a Greater Germany into reality. History and heart disease wait for no man, even *der Führer*.

CHAPTER 12

PARKINSONISM AND PARKINSON'S DISEASE

O f the illnesses that affected Adolf Hitler, the diagnoses of chronic irritable bowel syndrome and Parkinson's disease are the most universally accepted. Parkinson's disease is the second major medical problem that Hitler suffered during his lifetime. This neurological disorder shortened his life expectancy, reduced his ability to move, and was a constant reminder of his deteriorating health and impending death.

TYPES OF PARKINSONISM

To those who have studied Adolf Hitler's neurological problems, the physical findings of parkinsonism are undeniable. Less universal among neurologists, especially in the older literature, has been how best to categorize his motor findings among the various clinical varieties of parkinsonism. Because of this disagreement, some description of the possible types of parkinsonism seems warranted. These varieties include hysterical parkinsonism, drug-induced parkinsonism, post-encephalitic parkinsonism, and the most common form, that being so-called idiopathic Parkinson's disease.

Werner Maser in his 1973 book *Hitler: Legend, Myth and Reality* attributed Adolf Hitler's tremor that he dated to 1923 to a hysterical post-traumatic disorder. Maser believed Hitler's neurological abnormalities were a combat neurosis and resulted from Hitler having been gassed and wounded during World War I. While the possibility of a hysterical tremor exists for the 1923 tremor, it seems unlikely that Hitler's tremor would go away for two decades only to return, along with other motor findings such as gait abnormalities, movement anomalies, diminished facial expression, and changes in his handwriting. Maser's explanation of a hysterical tremor (abnormal psychological state that causes unexplained physical symptoms) seems a most unlikely explanation.

A second clinical variety relates to drug-induced parkinsonism. Leonard and Renate Heston wrote that Hitler's tremor might have resulted from methamphetamine treatment. While methamphetamine causes tremor, it gives rise to a different type of tremor from that seen with Parkinson's disease. The Hestons suggest, based on substantial research, that Hitler received methamphetamine (Vitamultin forte injections) from his personal physician, Morell. Indeed, dramatic and otherwise unexplained improvements in Hitler's exhausted state are described following these injections and are what would be expected following administration of methamphetamine.

According to Leonard Heston in his 1999 book *Medical Descent*, Professor Ernst-Günther Schenck, an inspector of nutrition for the SS, in 1943 surreptitiously had the Vitamultin forte analyzed. He ground up a gold-wrapped Vitamultin forte tablet and submitted it to a laboratory in the Nutrition Inspector's office (Vitamultin forte had a different wrapper to distinguish it from the usual Vitamultin preparation) and determined that it contained methamphetamine and caffeine in addition to vitamins. Later when Schenck provided his information to Heinrich Himmler, he was told to drop the matter and discuss it no further.

The Hestons correctly pointed out the well-known methamphetamine side effects of tremor and megalomania, and self-confidence beyond what the situation reasonably allows. They queried whether such a pharmaceutical effect might be seen in Hitler's impulsive and poorly thought-out military decisions, such as his decision to invade the Soviet Union. This questionable and ultimately disastrous decision according to the Hestons was made well prior to the German military becoming sufficiently prepared with its plans for advanced super weapons and still lacking in adequate stocks of standard munitions.

Certain inconsistencies arise with the Hestons attributing Hitler's tremor to methamphetamine use. The tremor that results from methamphetamine is a different type than with Parkinson's disease. The kind of tremor Hitler showed was slow three-to-five cycle/second tremor with the hand at rest and the fingers moving toward and away from the palm. In contrast, a methamphetamine induced tremor is a rapid side-to-side finger tremor of about twenty cycles/second appearing when the arms are outstretched or in action. The two types of tremor look nothing at all alike to an experienced examiner. Leonard Heston in his 2011 expanded book accepts Hitler's tremor and other findings as those of Parkinson's disease.

In fairness to the Hestons, they considered whether the process of making meth-amphetamine might somehow have been compromised during the war by a lack of proper chemicals and a breakdown in the usual pharmaceutical quality control procedures. They question if this might have resulted in an altered formulation that gave rise to a Parkinson's syndrome and a more typical Parkinson's tremor.

Such an outcome is not entirely out of the question. A 1983 issue of *Science* magazine by Dr. William Langston and others described a chemical shunting occurring in the overheated basement of an illicit drug manufacturer who was attempting to make a designer narcotic agent. Instead, the biochemist produced a compound that created in its young drug users a neurological illness that clinically looked identical to Parkinson's disease and responded in the same way to Parkinson's medicines.

Nevertheless, while this possibility is interesting, no available proof exists to support it in Hitler's case. Also, the chemical structure for opiates as referred to in Langston's article is far different than that for an amphetamine. This highly speculative hypothesis cannot be either confirmed or entirely disproved. While Fritz Redlich disputes the theory as being a viable contender for the cause of Adolf Hitler's parkinsonism, this possibility suffers mainly from a lack of hard evidence.

Another common form of parkinsonism encountered today is due to adverse effects of medicines. Best known causes for this variety are medicines that deplete the brain of the major neurotransmitter dopamine, such as reserpine (used years ago as an early treatment for high blood pressure) or that block the effects of dopamine in the brain, as do the so-called major tranquilizers. Nevertheless, reserpine and the major tranquilizers—Thorazine was the first to hit the market—were not synthesized until the early 1950s. It seems highly unlikely that Morell could have obtained these preparations, or that they even existed at the time Hitler suffered from his parkinsonism.

Other observers have suggested that Hitler had a third clinical variety of parkinsonism that resulted from the effects of encephalitis (so-called brain fever resulting from the Spanish flu). Beginning in 1917, a worldwide pandemic of encephalitis lethargica (referred to as von Economo's encephalitis or sleeping sickness) occurred. A small percentage of people who developed encephalitis developed a form of parkinsonism, particularly known for its muscular stiffness, strange and spasmodic uncontrollable eye movements (so-called oculogyric crises), and behavioral disturbances. While occasionally described with post-encephalitic parkinsonism, tremor was not a typical feature. It was believed during much of the early twentieth century that post-encephalitic parkinsonism was the only cause of parkinsonism. It is now recognized that many people who were not born until well after the pandemic later developed Parkinson's disease, disproving this earlier notion.

While this type of parkinsonism remains a consideration and has its supporters, the clinical descriptions of Hitler's neurological disorder and the available newsreel clips do not conform well to the clinical findings of post-encephalitic parkinsonism. The overall impression by most who have studied Adolf Hitler's neurological disorder supports an alternative diagnosis—idiopathic Parkinson's disease. This variety is the most common clinical variety of parkinsonism. This age-related neurological disorder, Parkinson's disease, typically begins in patients in their sixth decade, but may be seen as early as in the latter part of the second decade of life.

CLINICAL FEATURES OF IDIOPATHIC PARKINSON'S DISEASE

The constellation of movement-related symptoms and signs in idiopathic Parkinson's disease is well recognized and consists of slow movements (bradykinesia), a particular type of stiffness of the muscles (cogwheel rigidity), a slow resting hand tremor, handwriting difficulties, limited associated arm swing when walking, and staring type facial expression caused by infrequent blinking and widening of the distance between the upper and lower eyelids. In the more advanced condition balance problems and walking difficulties usually occur.

The stiffness of the muscles with Parkinson's disease can be felt by an examiner and is referred to as the cogwheeling variety of muscular stiffness. As the examiner moves the limb back and forth, he/she perceives intermittent catches in the muscle as if the muscle were caught on a cogwheel. Other features include diminished facial expression (so-called masked facial expression or hypomimia), soft speech (so-called hypophonia) and difficulty with articulation (so-called dysarthria), simian (ape-like) posturing of the hands (where the person walks with the back of the hands forward rather than the typical thumb forward position), and handwriting abnormalities (micrographia). These are all common features of idiopathic Parkinson's disease.

Depression is a common feature in Parkinson's disease and may often be a presenting symptom. Cognitive symptoms and signs appear late in many people with advanced disease. This important aspect of Parkinson's disease will be discussed in the next chapters, as it is believed to have affected Hitler's performance as chancellor and as the ultimate leader of Nazi Germany.

NON-MOTOR ASPECTS OF PARKINSON'S DISEASE

Some non-motor aspects also exist in many persons with Parkinson's disease. These symptoms and signs include oily seborrhea (an oiliness of the skin), dandruff (seborrheic dermatitis), depression often as a presenting symptom, muscular discomfort likely resulting from the increased muscular tone, tingling, numbness, pain, and constipation.

Despite the presence of non-motor symptoms and signs in many persons with Parkinson's disease, the diagnosis cannot be made without at least two of the three major features of the disorder (tremor, muscular stiffness, and slowness of movement). Since Parkinson's disease is a progressive neurological disorder, demonstration of progression is also often included in the diagnostic consideration.

CHAPTER 13

ONSET, FEATURES, AND TREATMENT OF HITLER'S PARKINSON'S DISEASE

Today someone diagnosed with Parkinson's disease can anticipate a near normal life expectancy, but this was not true in the pre-levodopa (L-dopa)—a medication used to treat Parkinson's disease—era in which Hitler lived. At the time Adolf Hitler developed Parkinson's disease, a person was expected to live an average of only eight to nine years following onset. As such, Parkinson's disease was, in Hitler's time, a killer.

Hitler's blank stare, his typical resting hand tremor, the cramped nature (micrographia) of his handwriting, his shuffling gait, his slowness of movement, and repeated descriptions of his soft and muffled voice all attest to his having developed the most common form of parkinsonism—idiopathic Parkinson's disease.

Toward the end of his life, Parkinson's disease made Hitler appear older than his years. According to the declassified report of Morris Leikind who worked in American intelligence during World War II, Dr. von Hasselbach, one of the most critical and reliable of Hitler's doctors, said, "Up until 1940 Hitler appeared to be much younger than he was. From that date he aged rapidly. . . . After 1943 he appeared to have grown old."

Authors and contacts of Hitler variably attributed the change in Hitler's appearance to his exhausted state, poor diet, lack of exercise, to the attempted assassination attempt via a bomb explosion in July 1944, and to overtreatment by Morell. In addition, historians have attributed his rapid aging to the stress of presiding over a losing war effort and his country bombed into ruins and rubble. Such catastrophes undoubtedly must have taken a physical and mental toll on Hitler.

In addition, however, a likely explanation for Hitler's apparent rapid aging was his advancing Parkinson's disease. Parkinson's disease is well known to advance the visual signs of aging. Playwrights and screenwriters have often used Parkinson's disease signs as a theatrical device for showing advancing age. Parkinson's disease does so by demonstrating the highly visual slowing of movements, stooped posture, stony facial expression, and trembling of the extremities. These features also visually suggest an aged individual.

DATING ONSET AND ITS IMPORTANCE

Determining the date of onset of Hitler's Parkinson's disease is important because of its predictable, late appearing and performance-impairing cognitive features. While dating the beginning of any chronic illness can prove difficult, Parkinson's disease, much more than others, readily reveals itself to visual observation. Hitler fortunately appeared in many newsreels, making careful inspection of him over the years much easier.

Video recordings are now used routinely to diagnose Parkinson's disease. While working from old newsreels is not as complete as performing a neurological examination (no such examination was ever documented), it provides a method frequently used today in telemedicine and in modern neurology to demonstrate the features of the various movement disorders.

The dating of the onset of Adolf Hitler's Parkinson's disease is important for determining its chronicity. As mentioned earlier, Werner Maser described a transient tremor in Hitler in 1923 during the Beer Hall Putsch, Hitler's unsuccessful attempt to overthrow the Bavarian government that resulted in his imprisonment for treason. This transient tremor was more likely an anxiety related tremor than the sort of tremor seen with idiopathic Parkinson's disease.

A more convincing argument for dating onset is Abraham Lieberman's 1997 contention in the journal *Movement Disorders*, a study based on 1933 newsreels showing Adolf Hitler's failure to swing his left arm when walking (a common presentation for Parkinson's disease). Adolf Hitler was forty-four years old in 1933.

Other writers date the onset of Adolf Hitler's Parkinson's disease to 1941 or 1942. During that time is when various non-neurologically trained associates noted the left-hand tremor and when Theodor Morell documented Hitler's left-hand tremor in his casebook. Morell believed the tremor to be hysteria, or of psychological origin. Nevertheless, Hitler's tremor was likely not his initial sign of Parkinson's disease, only the most obvious. While tremor is easily recognizable by people not well versed in Parkinson's disease, it frequently follows the less obvious onset of diminished arm swing, infrequent blinking, handwriting abnormalities, muscular stiffness, slow movement, or other more subtle signs of Parkinson's disease.

The significance of limited arm swing when diagnosing Parkinson's disease became vividly clear early on in my career as a neurologist. I recall the presenting complaint of a patient listed as "his self-winding watch has stopped." Indeed, the patient no longer had arm swing while walking sufficient to activate his self-winding watch. In that instance, only careful neurological examination revealed additional neurological signs that allowed a diagnosis of Parkinson's disease to be made in the absence of hand tremor.

In my experience as a neurologist, diminished arm swing when walking was often the first unrecognized sign of Parkinson's disease. In addition, rather than walking with a thumb forward positioning of the hand, the person with Parkinson's disease walks with the thumbs rotated inwardly. The back of the hand then faces forward, as it does with the great apes (so-called simian posturing). To a trained eye, this aspect of Parkinson's disease becomes easily observable, though it can be missed. In several instances I felt compelled to report my personally discomforting observation to friends in non-medical settings, who then sought out their physicians who confirmed the diagnosis and began beneficial treatment.

Some authors have mistakenly ascribed Hitler's lack of arm swing to an injury that he suffered during the Beer Hall Putsch. Hitler did suffer an injury to his shoulder blade, or in some accounts to his collarbone. Hitler later reported to one of his doctors that he had sustained a fracture of his left scapula that for a time limited the function of his arm. He later said he had over time regained full recovery from this injury.

While a fractured shoulder blade would have been painful, and for a time could explain a lack of associated arm swing when walking, newsreels after the 1923 Beer Hall Putsch and as late as 1943 demonstrated Hitler swinging his arm normally when walking. For this reason, attributing the lack of arm swing to old trauma fails to explain the inconsistent presentation of this symptom.

A 1934 snippet of newsreel shows what appears to be a tremor of his left hand during a Nuremberg rally. To an experienced eye, this clip, although brief, is fairly compelling evidence for a Parkinson's tremor.

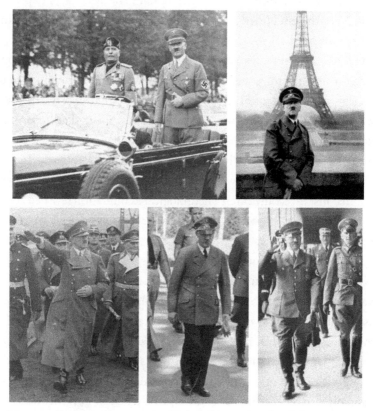

Montage of pictures demonstrating Hitler's characteristic hand placement utilized as a Parkinson's disease patient to control his embarrassing hand tremor. (Bundesarchiv, Bild 183-C13371, Bild 183-H12940, Bild 102-ow192A, Bild 146II-728, Bild 183-2006-0810-500, Bild 146-1977-149-13, US National Archives)

Many neurologists, including this author, have studied newsreels from later in Hitler's life and found convincing evidence for Parkinson's disease. These clips show the classic findings: stooped posture, short-stepped gait, slow pill-rolling type hand tremor, slowness of movement, and the typical stony facial expression.

HITLER'S HAND POSITIONING AND MICROGRAPHIA

Hitler's positioning of his left hand as seen in many newsreels is revealing. He adopted the mannerism of holding his left hand against his waist, gripping his belt, or fingering objects with his left hand. Newsreels often show him holding his gloves or a rolled piece of paper with his left hand. Hand placement, pressure on his belt, and finger manipulation of an object are common and useful methods that Parkinson's patients employ as a sensory trick to suppress their hand tremor.

I saw many patients in my practice with Parkinson's disease who revealed to me that they routinely would try to hide their tremor because it embarrassed them. Some patients while in public would hide their hands in their pockets or place the tremulous hand behind their backs. Others would resort to even sitting on the offending hand. Even more common was the sensory trick of involving the tremulous hand in some recurring activity such as playing with a coin, steadying the hand by holding onto an object, and even for short periods diminishing the tremor by sheer concentration.

One anecdote shared by another physician told of an outstanding neurosurgeon at a prestigious institution who had developed a Parkinson's tremor. While standing over a patient on the operating table with scalpel in his tremulous hand, the surgeon's hand would slowly descend toward the patient's brain. Just as the blade approached the surgical target, the scalpel would, as if by magic, stop oscillating, allowing the surgeon to make his precise incision or carry out another precise surgical technique. This striking visual image has stayed with me ever since learning of it, as it so graphically confirms the ability that intense concentration has in some patients to transiently stop their Parkinson's hand tremor.

Another characteristic clinical finding of Parkinson's disease seen with Hitler was his micrographia (literally small writing). This feature of Hitler's disease was for a long time either overlooked or misinterpreted. For example, Leikind in his World War II US intelligence summary attributed changes in Hitler's handwriting to "the uncertainty of old age," even though Hitler was only in his fifties.

Comparison of Adolf Hitler's signature from earlier in his life to that of the mid-1940s reveals dramatic changes that cover a spectrum from a normal signature to a strikingly micrographic one. Hitler's signature began to show the initial letter in the word written normally or somewhat smaller than normal, followed by a severe tapering off in size and legibility of the remaining letters. His signature progressively worsened and is typical of the micrographia of Parkinson's disease. Micrographia in Hitler's signature can arguably be seen as early as 1934 and clearly by 1937. By 1942 his signature became virtually illegible. By 1945 his signature looked like mere scratches on a page. At some point Hitler had to resort to using a stamped signature in place of his handwritten one.

From my own medical practice, I recall one patient with Parkinson's disease who became alarmed when his bank failed to recognize his micrographic signature and rejected his check. His signature had changed so considerably over the years that his micrographic signature aroused the bank's suspicion for potential fraud. Some

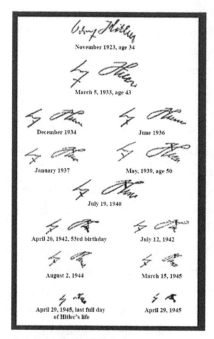

November 1923, age 34

March 5, 1933, age 43

December 1934

June 1936

January 1937

May, 1939, age 50

July 19, 1940

April 20, 1942, 53rd birthday

July 12, 1942

August 2, 1944

March 15, 1945

April 29, 1945, last full day of Hitler's life

April 29, 1945

A deterioration of Hitler's signature over time due to his Parkinson's disease. (Reprinted with permission of Abraham Lieberman, MD)

of my patients, recognizing the change in their signature and especially their slowness in signing checks, began routinely asking their spouses to write the checks. Such was particularly the case when trying to write a check at the checkout at the grocery store where often a line of impatient customers existed, waiting restlessly behind them. Other patients with Parkinson's disease would routinely write their checks minus the amount prior to visiting the store. Some would then ask the clerk at the cash register to add the amount for the purchase.

As mentioned previously, Morell did not recognize the signs of Parkinson's disease and was slow to document a diagnosis of Parkinson's disease in Hitler's medical casebook. Morell required outside assistance to help him recognize the nature of Hitler's tremor. Professor Walter Löhlein did precisely this, following an eye consultation performed on Hitler, and mentioned to Morell the likelihood of Hitler having Parkinson's disease. What exactly the eye doctor witnessed is unclear. Most likely Löhlein observed the slow resting tremor of Hitler's hand that predictably would have increased when Hitler felt emotional strain during the eye examination.

Löhlein apparently also passed this information to Professor Maximinus Friedrich Alexander de Crinis, a neurologist and psychiatrist as well as a high-ranking member of the SS, and who served with Löhlein on the faculty at the University of Berlin. Professor de Crinis had previously become suspicious that Hitler had developed Parkinson's disease from viewing newsreels of Hitler.

As a curious aside, de Crinis also wrote the Euthanasia Decree that was signed by Adolf Hitler on September 20, 1939. The Euthanasia Program brought about the systematic murder of institutionalized patients with physical or mental disabilities by using gas chambers. The program began with children but within two years was extended to adults. It preceded the genocide of European Jewry by approximately two years. When the war was lost, de Crinis, a fanatic Nazi, killed his family and himself by taking cyanide. It is also worth mentioning that Karl Brandt, one of Hitler's closest medical staff members and a colleague of de Crinis, directed the tragic Euthanasia Program.

As mentioned earlier, young Adolf was terrified of his schizophrenic aunt who lived with his family. The aunt's behavior was bizarre and inexplicable to the sensitive boy. Some authors have questioned whether this frightening childhood experience might have had an impact on Hitler's support for the Euthanasia Program in which de Crinis and Brandt were heavily involved.

This information regarding de Crinis's suspicion of Hitler having Parkinson's disease was relayed back to Morell and may have further prompted Morell to belatedly diagnose Parkinson's disease (paralysis agitans as it was known in those days). Morell soon began treatment for the tremor with something other than the showy but ineffective electrotherapy he had introduced earlier for treatment of Hitler's tremor. Morell recorded the diagnosis of paralysis agitans for "Patient A" in Hitler's medical file in early 1945.

A 1945 newsreel by Swedish media escaped German censorship. This clip was made at a time toward the end of World War II when Nazi censorship was breaking down. This newsreel represents conclusive evidence for Hitler's Parkinson's disease by demonstrating a coarse, slow, resting tremor of the left hand, lack of a normal facial expression, and demonstrates a stooped posture and short, shuffling steps—all unmistakable and diagnostic features for Parkinson's disease. This clip is diagnostic in and of itself for Parkinson's disease.

In summary, the features of Hitler's Parkinson's disease are clear. The date of the onset of his neurological illness is likely 1933 or 1934 based on his lack of arm swing. Also, a second sign of Parkinson's disease was likely present in 1934 and certainly evident in 1937 in his micrographic handwriting of his signature. Both lack of arm swing and micrographia long predate Morell's documentation and the observations of others regarding the appearance of Hitler's hand tremor.

TREATMENT OF HITLER'S PARKINSON'S DISEASE

Surprisingly and inadvertently, Hitler received treatment that likely reduced his tremor. For his chronic gastrointestinal bloating and flatulence, Hitler for years had taken Dr. Koester's anti-gas pills. This treatment contained belladonna, which is known to reduce tremors. Similar belladonna-like agents are still used in a limited fashion even today in the treatment of Parkinson's disease. Belladonna-like agents were the mainstay of treatment for Parkinson's disease before the advent of L-dopa in the mid-1960s.

For only the last two weeks of Hitler's life, Morell prescribed Homberg 680, a belladonna-like medicine that was only used to treat Parkinson's disease. He started this medicine with an upward tapering schedule of drops taken by mouth. Morell also began giving Hitler subcutaneous injections of Harmin, also a belladonna-like agent.

In retrospect, it makes no sense whatsoever to begin two such agents at the same time for treatment of Hitler's tremor, yet such prescriptive practices were altogether typical for the therapeutic enthusiast Dr. Theodor Morell.

In summary, Adolf Hitler suffered from idiopathic Parkinson's disease that began as early as 1933 or 1934 according to Abraham Lieberman, a prominent American neurologist and authority on Parkinson's disease. Lieberman based this dating on Hitler's lack of associated arm swing when walking. Reviewing Hitler's signature also reveals the well accepted findings of micrographia and further dates the onset of Hitler's Parkinson's disease to well prior to the often mistakenly accepted date of 1941.

This neurological disorder in Hitler's time was without effective treatment and a person with this disorder could be expected to live only about eight to nine years following its onset. Hitler would not have been expected to live beyond the early to mid-1940s, a shortening of his life expectancy independent from his coronary artery heart disease, which in and of itself decreased life expectancy.

Adolf Hitler must have felt as if he were living on borrowed time. It is likely he possessed a sense of urgency to carry out his military plans to achieve his lifelong goal of *Lebensraum* before being overtaken by his illnesses. Following his death, other German leaders could then successfully manage the ongoing affairs of state. Hitler's egoism, megalomania, and narcissism pushed him to complete his lifelong dream of a Greater Germany, a Germany free from what he considered the Jewish/Bolshevik scourge.

CHAPTER 14

BEHAVIORAL CHANGES WITH ADVANCED PARKINSON'S DISEASE

T he movement features of Parkinson's disease are well known and have been since the original 1817 description of "the shaking palsy" by the Englishman, Dr. James Parkinson. The physical characteristics were also known in antiquity, but the neurobehavioral effects of chronic Parkinson's disease have received attention only in the last thirty years. This chapter will review the cognitive changes now known to be associated with chronic Parkinson's disease. A second behavioral change associated with Parkinson's disease, a sleep disturbance, will be discussed as it too may have affected Adolf Hitler.

COGNITIVE IMPAIRMENT

In 1996 V. Soukup and R. L. Adams determined (as have other neuropsychologists) that the most reliably found cognitive impairment with Parkinson's disease consists of difficulty with concept formation, sequence planning, shifting and maintaining sets, and temporal ordering. In other words, people with chronic Parkinson's disease have difficulty shifting from one thought to another and in breaking away from old ideas and forming newer ones. This disorder manifests as mental rigidity and inflexibility. In neuropsychological terms, this syndrome is called a disorder of executive function.

These findings, in neurological terms, describe what is known neurologically as a type of frontal lobe syndrome. In contrast to the better-known Alzheimer's disease, Parkinson's disease does not have the wide array of cognitive symptoms as does Alzheimer's disease and is usually not very apparent to casual observers. The milder frontal lobe dysfunction in advanced Parkinson's disease may even escape notice by family and close friends but still give rise to debilitating cognitive abnormalities when the person attempts to deal with matters involving complexity. The detection of Parkinson's behavioral changes may even require careful neuropsychological testing.

Based on historical information, my colleagues and I in 1999 first described these neuropsychological losses in Adolf Hitler. A study by Matthew Lambert and Janet Schwantz from our Parkinson's disease center demonstrated that patients who had Parkinson's disease for ten years or longer demonstrated this type of executive dysfunction.

Authenticating the duration of Parkinson's disease for Adolf Hitler proves important for predicting his cognitive function. At the time of the Battle of Normandy and the Battle of the Bulge, based on Abraham Lieberman's dating from lack of arm swing, Hitler would have had Parkinson's disease for more than the ten critical years. This conclusion, based on duration of Parkinson's signs, is also further supported by historical observations from Hitler's colleagues.

HISTORICAL EVIDENCE FOR HITLER'S COGNITIVE IMPAIRMENT

Interrogations of high-ranking Nazi officials following World War II provided valuable information regarding Hitler's cognitive dysfunction caused by Parkinson's disease. Professor Carl Eichen, who treated Hitler, revealed in his interrogation the following: "His [Hitler's] movements and reactions, both physical and mental, had become slower and he now trembled frequently."

Ear, nose, and throat doctor Erwin Giesing recalled how in September 1944, Hitler's hand shook so badly that he had to put it down on the desk and wait awhile before dashing off his signature in one scratchy flourish. Giesing commented on how the tremor had advanced to his right side by the autumn of 1944 (Irving, *The Secret Diaries of Hitler's Doctor*). Since Hitler was right-handed, this observation by Giesing confirmed the disease by that time involved both sides of his body.

According to Percy Ernst Schramm, Colonel-General Heinz Guderian, who was an early proponent of Blitzkrieg, referred to Hitler's mental inflexibility in Irving's book by saying: "In February 1945, Hitler seemed absent-minded and unable to concentrate. He was exhausted and could barely move around. He still sensed the essence of contradictory reports but had lost his mental flexibility and

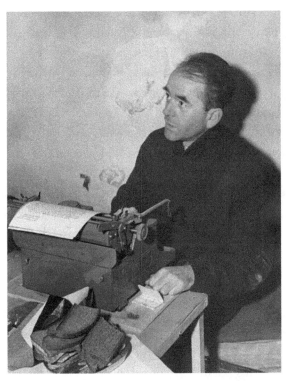

Albert Speer, friend and confidant of Adolf Hitler and the last resident of Spandau prison. (United States Army Signal Corps, 1945, Harvard Law School Library, Harvard University, Hollis Collection)

imagination." It is hard to imagine a clearer and more concise description of this neuropsychological syndrome than what is credited to General Guderian.

Albert Speer in his foreword to Leonard and Renate Heston's book, *Adolf Hitler: A Medical Descent That Changed History*, also described changes in Hitler's behavior. Extractions from Speer's 1953 notes characterized Hitler in 1938 as having allowed his associates to take full responsibility for their assigned fields and having accepted their conclusions without further examination. As time progressed, Hitler changed and began to avoid collaborative discussions, making decisions based solely on his own views. Hitler seemingly became besotted by his own opinions and impervious to the judgments of others. The German General Staff is viewed historically as having performed well in the early part of World War II when Hitler readily delegated to his trusted advisors. Later in the war, however, Hitler did not delegate well, which reduced the effectiveness of his top military leaders and the overall success rate of the German forces.

From the summer of 1942 onward, it struck Speer how rigid Hitler had become in his thinking. He described Hitler's mind moving along an "unalterable track." Speer described Hitler at this stage of his life as showing a "dull obstinacy . . . [c]learly having lost the mental agility of his earlier days. He lacked the capacity for thinking through large-scale conceptualizations, instead focusing on more trivial matters that should have been delegated to his, by then, frustrated generals." These observations collectively and convincingly provide descriptions of major changes in Hitler's behavior and strongly suggest the typical cognitive impairment that is now known to exist with chronic Parkinson's disease.

At a time when Hitler was planning or executing major troop movements and strategy, the pathology of his Parkinson's disease was staging its own march throughout his brain. The disease moved relentlessly through Hitler's undefended brainstem and, later by way of subcortical pathways, outflanked his frontal lobes. The behavioral changes of Parkinson's disease, combined with Hitler's stubborn, paranoid, grandiose, and narcissistic personality, impaired his once crisp decision-making. Hitler's altered behavior and lack of delegation also reduced the effective workings of his General Staff. This deterioration in his mental abilities led to serious delays in issuing timely orders and gave rise to egregious errors in dispensing and carrying out military plans.

SLEEP DISTURBANCES

In addition to Hitler's neuropsychological changes, sleep disturbances existed in Hitler as they do for many people with Parkinson's disease. Of course, poor quality sleep can further reduce the quality of life and impair mental performance. Surprisingly, sleep abnormalities were even mentioned in the original 1817 description by James Parkinson.

The usual patterns of deep and restful sleep are often diminished with Parkinson's disease, especially with advanced disease. It takes longer for a person to fall asleep, and the quality of the sleep is less restful. The sleep architecture changes with the typical long periods of deep and restful sleep becoming disrupted with increased awakenings, causing the sleep to be less refreshing. As a result, the person with Parkinson's disease feels less rested on waking and often suffers from excessive daytime sleepiness. Such sleepiness further impairs mental clarity and cognitive performance.

It is believed that such a disturbance in Hitler existed, affecting his sleep/wake cycle, as he was well known to have unusual sleep habits. The significance of this aspect of his health will be addressed later in the context of the Battle of Normandy.

CHAPTER 15

IMPACT OF HITLER'S FAILING HEALTH

ENCROACHING INFIRMITIES

Keeping in mind the life-shortening effects of Hitler's heart and brain disorders, a brief review of his encroaching infirmities and their potential for impacting his decision-making is in order. Hitler must have been aware at some level of his diminishing movements. Even if he did not know the name for his medical infirmity, he must have realized his loss of dexterity and slowed physical movements.

When working with persons with Parkinson's disease I daily heard complaints about difficulty tying shoelaces, operating a keyboard or typewriter, counting small change, shaving, combing hair, and multiple other aspects of everyday life and personal hygiene. It surprised me when my patients shared the exaggerated length of time that it took them to get out of bed in the morning, shower or wash up, get dressed, and prepare for their day ahead. Routinely for persons with Parkinson's disease this length of time would be doubled or tripled compared to pre-Parkinson's disease days. As driven a man as Hitler was, such difficulties must have been galling and hugely frustrating for him.

It is also highly likely that Hitler was aware of his coronary artery disease, his abnormal electrocardiograms, and their prediction for his diminished life expectancy. As previously stated, Hitler had always obsessed over his symptoms and illnesses and would likely have demanded explanations from Morell and queried his doctor as to why he needed repeated electrocardiograms.

Additionally, Hitler's family history of shortened life expectancy led him to believe that he would not live to old age. On occasion following a strategic planning session, Hitler would mention to the participants in the session that he

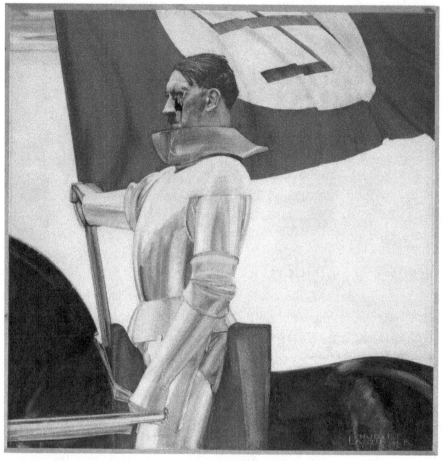

Propaganda poster of a noble-appearing Hitler astride a horse as the standard-bearer of Nazism. (Reprinted with permission of Erich Lessing/Art Resource, NY)

might not live long enough to see the outcome of the plans under consideration. Hitler's doctors understood the prognosis in the 1930s and 1940s for someone individually with Parkinson's disease and for coronary artery disease. They also would have recognized that the combination of these two major illnesses would shorten Hitler's life even further.

QUESTIONS REGARDING TIMING FOR THE INVASION OF THE SOVIET UNION

The principal reasons behind the timing of Germany's attack on the Soviet Union in 1941 have been much debated and will be discussed at length in the next chapter. However, the dual-pronged rationale of the German Nazi Party was the removal

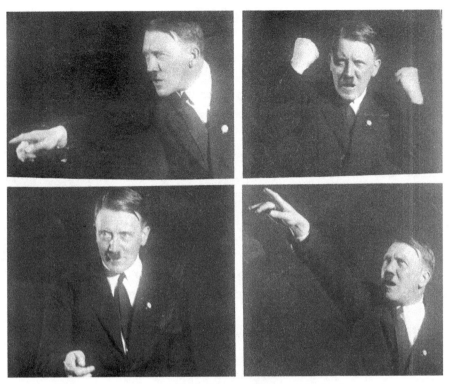

Hitler practicing his gesticulations in front of a mirror. He was said to be the preeminent orator of the twentieth century, with a mesmerizing effect on the war-weary German people. (Bundesarchiv, Bild 102-10640)

of the indigenous Jews and Slavs and the acquisition of *Lebensraum*. While these core factors predicted the inevitability of a war between Germany and Russia, they did not determine the timing of this huge and pivotal military misadventure.

FAILING HEALTH IN HITLER—THE ARYAN ICON

Adolf Hitler began serving as Germany's supreme leader in 1934. The Nazi Party, through a massive propaganda campaign, encouraged the citizenry of Germany to view him in God-like terms. Hitler was an egoist and along with Germany's Nazi Party wished to epitomize the so-called Aryan race.

Hitler was the first German politician to routinely use an airplane to campaign. Propaganda at the time capitalized on his modern flair and utilized heroic symbolism to enhance Hitler's image. Through his clever verbal and visual propaganda, Goebbels polished this larger-than-life, God-like image of Hitler.

Imagine the blow to Hitler's self-image when later he began to spill food on his clothing from his shaking hand, encountered difficulty tying his shoelaces, and experienced clumsiness when retrieving coins or pens from his pocket. His all too human foibles must have given rise to great consternation.

Not only did his Parkinson's disease affect his movements, but it also changed his speech. At his peak in the early 1930s, Adolf Hitler may have been the greatest orator of the twentieth century. He had a hypnotic verbal persuasiveness that when combined with his well-practiced gesticulations and piercing gaze added immensely to his personal magnetism.

As his Parkinson's disease progressed, however, Hitler's public appearances by necessity became less frequent. Joseph Goebbels gave most of the speeches during the last years of the war. Hitler's absence from the public eye resulted from his Parkinson's disease, as his hard-to-miss hand tremor proved increasingly difficult to disguise.

Albert Speer in *Inside the Third Reich* described Adolf Hitler toward the end of the war in unmistakably parkinsonian terms. Speer confirmed the progression of Hitler's Parkinson's disease by describing him as follows:

> His limbs trembled; he walked stooped with dragging footsteps. Even his voice became quavering and lost its old masterfulness. Its force had given way to a faltering, toneless manner of speaking . . . his uniform which in the past he had kept scrupulously neat, was often neglected in the last period of his life and stained by the food he had eaten with a shaking hand.

David Irving in *The Secret Diaries of Hitler's Doctor* provided a description of Hitler given in the autumn of 1944 by Field Marshal Gerd von Rundstedt. Rundstedt described Hitler's posture as stooped and that he trembled with both arms, the right more so than the left. He also noted that Hitler was becoming lost in the details of his military briefings.

Dr. Karl Brandt, Hitler's personal surgeon, also noticed that Hitler's memory was failing him. Hitler was having difficulty following conversations, was "flighty," and rambled on about inconsequential matters. These failings were increasingly problematic for those serving on Hitler's General Staff.

Volker Ullrich in his 2020 book *Hitler's Downfall, 1930–1945* provided further descriptions of a deteriorating Hitler. Ullrich quoted Goebbels saying in early 1945, "It chokes me up to see the *Führer* in his bunker in such a withered condition." Other observers noticed his face looked paler and more like a mask than normal, his physical tremor had worsened, his movements were lamer, and he stooped more.

Cavalry Cpt. Gerhard Boldt noted that "his handshake was limp and soft, without any strength and making no impression. His head bobbled slightly. . . . His left arm dangled lamely, and his left hand shook badly. . . . All of his movements were those of an ill, senile man. He reminded me of a burned-out piece of iron."

Fritz Redlich described Hitler's deterioration as being apparent even to lay people. Gauleiter Karl Wahl (a party functionary) described on February 24, 1945:

> Hitler talked, sitting at a table for about an hour and a half. His voice was not very loud. Sitting very close in the second or third row I could observe him in minute detail. . . . Then I really perceived what a bad state of health he was in. His left hand, or rather his left arm shook so badly and constantly that the whole body began to vibrate. This was not trembling; these were strong and regular shaking movements, which disquieted me greatly during the speech. Whatever he undertook to suppress these movements, which were apparently embarrassing for him, he did not succeed. When he crossed his arms over his chest it got worse, the whole upper torso started to move.

During the final five years of his life, Hitler's public appearances became constrained, and films and newsreels prior to their release required careful censoring to delete the most obvious signs of Parkinson's disease. Keeping in mind how Parkinson's disease appears to age a person, what an anathema for the supreme leader of the Third Reich to be so enfeebled. What a shock it would have been had the German nation known that Hitler was no Superman, but instead was a prematurely aging, frail, and tremulous mortal.

In 1941 Hitler would have had Parkinson's disease for eight years. By this time a patient's independence for daily tasks such as dressing and hygiene, walking, and balance is typically reduced. In addition, the voice of a person with eight years of disease might also become soft and muffled and the patient's face would develop a lack of expression and reduced blink rate, causing a staring type of facial expression (referred to in neurological terms as hypomimia). By 1941 Hitler's symptoms would have advanced to the point that his physical activities would have been limited. While Hitler would have likely known his prognosis, the German people were still ignorant of it. His visually apparent illness made sustaining his image especially challenging.

Recall also that Hitler had worsening electrocardiograms and was under treatment for "coronary sclerosis." Hypertension, a cause for stroke and heart attacks, was present. In those days no treatment was provided for high blood pressure and no truly effective treatment was known that reduced the progression of coronary artery disease. Since heart disease was understood to shorten lives, Hitler likely felt his death to be not far off. Every time he suffered chest pain he would have been reminded of his limited life expectancy. As a result of his poor prognosis from both Parkinson's disease and heart disease, if Hitler was to gain *Lebensraum* for Germany and overthrow Stalin's communist government, time was rapidly running out for him.

While the German military might have been stronger several years after 1941—perhaps in 1944 when the Molotov-Ribbentrop Pact was due to expire—Hitler's mental and physical capabilities would predictably have been diminished, and he might not even survive that long. At the Berghof conference on August 22, 1939, Hitler stressed to the planners the need to attack the Soviet Union. According to David Gompert, Hans Binnendijk, and Bonny Lin: "There is no time to lose. War must come in *my lifetime* [emphasis added by author]. My pact [Molotov/Ribbentrop] was meant only to stall for time, and gentlemen, to Russia will happen just what I have practiced with Poland—we will crush the Soviet Union."

In addition to military arguments, the question of Hitler's life expectancy and his centrality to the Nazi ideals must also be considered as factors in the timing of Operation Barbarossa. Hitler's imminent mortality and egoism, grandiose narcissism, and hatred of the Bolshevik state influenced his decision to invade the Soviet Union in June 1941.

This invasion would prove to be a huge strategic blunder and was a major factor in the outcome of World War II. With the benefit of hindsight, we know this decision was disastrous for the German cause. The opportunity for German success several years later, when the German-Soviet pact ended, is a matter of ongoing debate, but it is doubtful that the outcome for Nazi Germany could have been any worse.

CHAPTER 16

OPERATION BARBAROSSA

Hitler renamed the invasion of the Soviet Union Operation Barbarossa. He took this codename from Frederick I who was king of Germany from 1153 to 1190 and Emperor of the Holy Roman Empire from 1155 to 1190. This codename replaced earlier operation plan names, including Operation Fritz, as given by Lt. Col. Bernhard von Lossberg, and Operation Otto, as given by Gen. Franz Halder.

ARGUMENTS FOR AND AGAINST THE LAUNCHING OF OPERATION BARBAROSSA IN 1941

Ian Kershaw in his 1998 biography of Hitler describes Hitler's growing belief in 1940 and 1941 that Russia was the key to removing England from the war. Volker Ullrich in his 2020 book *Hitler's Downfall, 1930–1945* described Hitler's belief that England's great hope was Russia and America: "If the hope in Russia is gone, the same will be true in America because the Russian disappearance will lead to a tremendous bolstering of Japan's status in the Far East." So long as Russia existed, Kershaw wrote, England maintained hope for Russian assistance and therefore obdurately remained in the war.

Hitler maintained that this prop for keeping Great Britain in the war had to be removed. A defeated Russia would further demoralize England and would allow Germany to pit additional forces against this small but stubbornly resistant island nation. Also, a German attack on Russia would require a shift of Soviet troops staged against Japan in the Far East, allowing Japan to redeploy its own forces to areas of greater concern to the United States. Orienting the United States toward the Pacific War would have been a positive step, thought Hitler, according to both Kershaw and Ullrich.

In April and May 1941, Stalin purged many of his most capable Soviet officers. Hitler saw this as an auspicious opportunity since this expulsion weakened the effectiveness of the Soviet military. This reorganization resulted from poor performance on behalf of various officers and units and arguably resulted as well from Stalin's paranoia. In any event, Hitler saw Russia as weakened, but a vulnerability that would not last for long. This purging of the Soviet military may have accelerated Hitler's plans for an early invasion.

Germany depended on the Soviet Union for raw materials that were vital for its ongoing war effort. Hitler did not believe the flow of these valuable resources would continue indefinitely. He viewed the Soviet diplomatic policies as hardening against Germany, ultimately resulting in the reduction in the flow of natural resources from Russia to Greater Germany. Hitler wanted to directly control these necessary resources by way of invasion and occupation.

The growing industrial and military strength of the United States was also becoming an increasing concern for Hitler. The US had begun to rearm and to assist Great Britain by supplying needed armaments and raw materials. In March 1941 the passage of the Lend-Lease Act indicated to Hitler the importance that the US held for maintaining Great Britain in the war. Kershaw describes that Hitler correctly understood the intentions of the American government and its hostility to the interests of the German Reich.

Stephen Fritz in his 2018 book *First Soldier: Hitler as a Military Leader* suggests that following the Munich Agreement in 1938, British Prime Minister Neville Chamberlain believed Germany too weak economically and militarily to launch a war, while Hitler believed Germany had a dwindling military advantage that could be lost to a rearming Britain.

These factors collectively are believed by many World War II historians to have favored Hitler beginning the war against the Soviet Union in 1941. In addition, little evidence exists that the German High Command, at least in public, differed materially from Hitler's opinion. If indeed the German High Command had reservations, most of the military leaders did not directly voice them to Hitler. However, they repeatedly voiced their reservations to each other in private.

Ullrich makes the important point that the final decision for war with Russia came from Hitler. Hitler had increasingly grown into his job as overall commander-in-chief following German success against France and England. While listening to his generals and maintaining his military options for as long as possible, Hitler maintained control over final decision-making.

In addition to these military and economic factors, the timing of Hitler's decision to launch Operation Barbarossa is believed by the current author to have been influenced by his failing health, though the German High Command would have understood none of these health concerns. Nevertheless, the worsening of Hitler's performance and his diminished life expectancy created for Hitler a sense of urgency that he might not live long enough to assure Germany's dominance on the world stage.

Robert Waite claims that Hitler's decision to go to war two years earlier in September 1939 resulted from his fear of getting old. In a major speech to his military commanders in August 1939 Hitler spoke of the need for war by saying, "I don't have time to wait. . . . I can't lose a single year. I've got to get to power shortly to solve the gigantic problems during the time remaining for me. I have got to. I have got to." And on another occasion, "I need ten years of lawmaking. The time is short. I have not long enough to live." Keeping in mind that Hitler was only fifty years old when he said this, hardly on the doorstep of senescence, Hitler probably had in mind his progressive illnesses and knowledge of his limited long-term effectiveness.

The unleashing of Operation Barbarossa in June 1941 ultimately proved unsuccessful and ended up being a very poor decision. The invasion occurred prior to Germany's production of its qualitatively superior instruments of warfare (its so-called wonder weapons) or even having filled its stockpiles of conventional arms.

While Germany had earlier considered long-range bombers that would have benefitted the invasion (and would have been useful for bombing England), they did not delay the invasion to allow for reconsideration of this vital need. Few would dispute that Germany would have been stronger militarily three years hence. The question exists as to whether Germany's enemies would also have been stronger in 1944, thus providing some historians with arguments against delaying the invasion of the Soviet Union.

Other issues should have been addressed prior to the German invasion as well, such as how to adequately resupply the invading German forces and how to solve the problem of differing railway gauge between Germany and the Soviet Union. Germany's poor military intelligence regarding Soviet munitions and especially its number of tanks, abetted by German hubris over the adequacy of Soviet troops and their leadership, provided overconfidence among Hitler's German High Command, all of which compounded logistical issues.

PLANNING OPERATION BARBAROSSA

Between January and March 1941 and under maximum security, the operational plans for Operation Barbarossa were finalized. Hitler approved these plans. But even earlier Hitler speaking to the Reichstag on January 30, 1939, had linked the coming invasion to a broader general war on Jewry. Hitler painted a picture of a war of either annihilation or deportation of the Jews and Slavs to allow *Lebensraum* for a Greater Germany. According to Kershaw the idea of destroying the Jews once and for all was just beginning to take shape in Hitler's mind.

Planning for the military invasion was largely under the direction of OKH (Army High Command). Gen. Franz Halder along with army Commander-in-Chief Walther von Brauchitsch, who had earlier orchestrated the successful invasion of Poland. Both played major roles in planning Operation Barbarossa.

Halder and the Army High Command held that the principal objective of the campaign should be to capture the Soviet capital, Moscow. This was classical military doctrine as per Carl von Clausewitz. Hitler on the other hand preferred capturing Leningrad along with Ukraine, the breadbasket of the Soviet Union, as well as the oil fields in the Caucasus. By doing so Hitler held that the German forces would starve the Soviet Union of both fuel and foodstuffs. Stalin and his generals suspected the plan as put forth by Hitler to be the more likely. Hitler also envisioned the northern and southern attacking forces serving as a giant pincer movement that would capture huge numbers of Soviet soldiers and vast amounts of Soviet armament.

Halder and Hitler clashed repeatedly over the formulation of the strategic goals and other details of the Barbarossa plan. Halder held that Moscow could be captured before the onset of winter, a prediction that turned out to be very wrong. His belief that capturing an adversary's capital would end the war was of course a long-standing military doctrine. Nevertheless, the plan adopted and agreed to by Hitler added the objective of capturing Moscow along with capturing Russia's key energy resources, food supplies, and Leningrad. The vast geography on which the campaign was to be fought, the huge resources necessary for military success, and an early Russian winter presaged the defeat of the German forces.

GERMAN MILITARY DISAGREEMENT

In *The Memoirs of Field Marshal Wilhelm Keitel,* the Chief of the Wehrmacht High Command (OKW) noted that Hitler's decision to prepare for war with the Soviet Union was made in early December 1940 but the planning had been initiated the summer before. Hitler's determination to invade the Soviet Union and its timing shocked Keitel and was made over the latter's strenuous objections.

Field Marshal Keitel's responsibilities lay in infrastructure, armament, personnel, and other bureaucratic tasks, all of which were vital for German military success. He believed such matters to be of little interest to Hitler. Hitler preferred to focus on tactics and operational details that lay within the realm of the OKH (Army High Command), and he often ignored input from Keitel who was with the OKW (Wehrmacht High Command). Keitel knew well the status of armaments and personnel and he held that Germany was unprepared for Operation Barbarossa and believed the invasion unnecessary.

GERMANY LACKED WONDER WEAPONS

In addition to lacking sufficient personnel and adequate stocks of standard military equipment in 1941, many of Germany's qualitatively superior weapons of war had not yet become fully available. The German sound-activated torpedoes, V-1 and V-2 rockets, and jet-propelled airplanes (the Me-261 jet fighter and the Arado Blitz bomber) were not slated for full-scale production until later.

Questions arise among historians as to whether the presence of these newer and qualitatively superior German weapons of war would have brought about a different outcome for Operation Barbarossa. We now know that the launching of Operation Barbarossa beginning in June 1941 was a drastic failure and a clear turning point in World War II. Whether or not the Allies would have matched the Germans in the production of more modern weapons of war during the next three years cannot be determined with certainty. Likewise, whether the United States would have in the interim sufficiently ramped up its huge industrial output in support of the Allies remains arguable. Clearly Roosevelt wished to assist Great Britain, but domestic politics tended to limit the extent of the support the United States could offer. In any event the delay by Germany until Hitler's "wonder weapons" were available did not occur.

Let's briefly review some of the qualitatively superior German instruments of warfare. The German military knew full well that Germany would be outnumbered and outgunned. All along Hitler and his General Staff depended on qualitatively superior weaponry, improved military tactics, and better trained and more disciplined troops. Toward this end aircraft played an important role.

To the detriment of the Germany military preparedness between 1939 and 1941 according to the Warfare History Network, Hitler informed the German aeronautical industry of new restrictions on aircraft research and development. But by 1942 Hitler and his Air Force High Command had changed their collective mind due to the German Messerschmitt M-109 fighter having lost ground to the newer Allied long-range fighters, such as the North American P-51 Mustang.

The constant bombardment of Germany and other Axis powers by Allied Air Forces compelled Hitler to invest in newer airplane technology. It was at that time that the German aircraft industry rushed to build the world's first operational jet fighter—the Messerschmitt Me-262. This airplane first flew in May 1943 and was described by its test pilot as "like being pushed by angels." With a speed of more than 540 miles per hour, the jet plane was at least 150 miles an hour faster than any Allied warplane, though the aircraft suffered from poor maneuverability. The jet fighter had a ceiling of 37,565 feet and had a range of 652 miles. Despite these remarkable features, Hitler again slowed the development of the plane in 1943 due to concerns over its great fuel consumption, only then to rush it back into development in early 1944.

Despite its design as a fighter, Hitler decreed that the Me-262 would be used as a bomber. In part this decision may have resulted from its relative lack of maneuverability. But Hitler wanted the Me-262 jet fighter-bomber to exact a fitting retribution on England for the nearly constant bombing that Germany had suffered.

In contrast to the Me-262, the Arado Blitz bomber was designed from the beginning as a jet bomber. It was a revolutionary aircraft that may have impacted the course of the war had it arrived in service earlier. While it had been planned from 1941 onward, the prototype did not make its appearance until June 1943. A year later two types of Blitz bombers entered the war: the Arado Ar 234B-1 in January 1945, and the Arado Ar 234B-2 that became the principal production model. It flew at a top speed of 461 miles per hour, ceiling of 32,810 feet, and a range of 1,103 miles. Its bomb load was 3,300 pounds.

The German sound-activated torpedo was another German technological advance and was deployed to a limited extent by German U-boats during World War II. A forerunner of the G-7 torpedo was introduced in March 1943 but had only been fired by three U-boats by September of that year. Both Jak Showell in his 2009 work *Hitler's Navy: A Reference Guide to the Kreigsmarine* and John Campbell in his 1985 book *Naval Weapons of World War II* provide background on this novel naval advance. The G-7 was faster, had greater range, and possessed a magnetic exploder. It employed a passive acoustic homing system to find its target, meaning the technology homed in on the noise generated by the surface ship's propeller.

When in 1943 the Allied intelligence services learned of this German advance in torpedo technology, they immediately began to develop countermeasures including acoustic decoys. Again, this advanced and qualitatively superior technology came too late to have brought about a major impact on the war.

The question again arises, had the German technology been kept under wraps for several more years, would the German U-boat onslaught in the Atlantic that proved so vital to both England and the Soviet Union been sufficiently effective to impact later developments in the war?

Additional so-called "wonder weapons" included the German V-2 guided missile and the small pilotless aircraft known as the flying bomb or V-1. The early models of the V-2 were produced by 1939, but Hitler felt the program was unneeded. Only later when the Luftwaffe lost the Battle of Britain was the rocket program given full approval. After several failed launches, a successful launch in 1942 convinced Hitler and his Luftwaffe advisors to pursue its development.

The V-2 carried a one-ton payload and was fired from a location around The Hague in the Netherlands. Hitler realized the weapon's great potential and ordered it mass-produced. Initially the V-2 launched from concrete launching pads but eventually was fitted on mobile launching devices. These mobile launching pads could be camouflaged, making them difficult for the Allied warplanes to locate and attack. The V-2s reached a speed of 3,580 miles per hour with a range of 200 miles. Just four minutes after takeoff, the V-2 could come crashing down on London. Hitler saw this weapon as a vengeance weapon that instilled fear within his enemies.

The V-1 or flying bomb also offered Hitler a way of retaliating for the nearly constant bombardment that Germany had suffered. The flying bomb flew along a preset gyroscopic-controlled course. While lacking accuracy, it was sufficiently accurate to hit London. Because of technical issues the V-1 did not become fully operational until the summer of 1944 when 5,000 operational V-1s were in place for use against London.

The question remains as to whether the German rocketry program would have had a substantial effect on the outcome of the war had it been stockpiled and used later. Would the Allied defenses several years later have been substantially altered to have countered this German advance? Such hypothetical questions cannot be answered with any degree of certainty.

Unfortunately for Germany's cause, these later dates for full implementation of Hitler's "wonder weapons" as we have seen did not mesh well with Hitler's concerns about his own survival.

Keitel later held in his own defense before the Nuremberg Tribunal that he had tried to dissuade Hitler from launching the attack on the USSR. He based his argument on the grounds that it was an unnecessary war, as Germany already

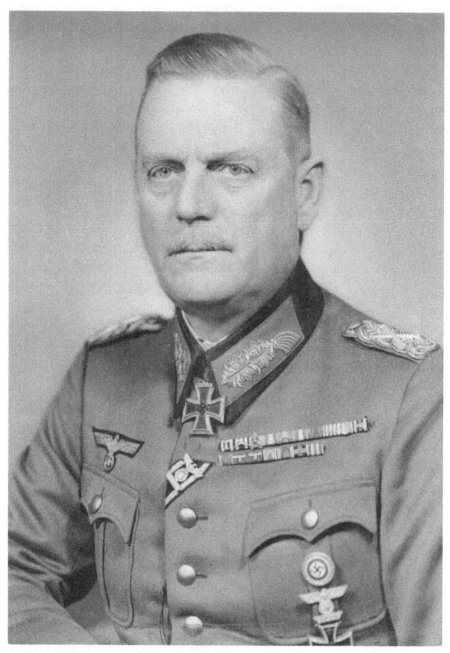

Field Marshal Wilhelm Keitel. (Bundesarchiv, Bild 183-H30220)

benefitted from its semi-alliance with the Soviet Union. Keitel also argued that it was clear to him that the offensive against the Soviet Union would overextend the German military personnel and matériel capabilities. Keitel felt that

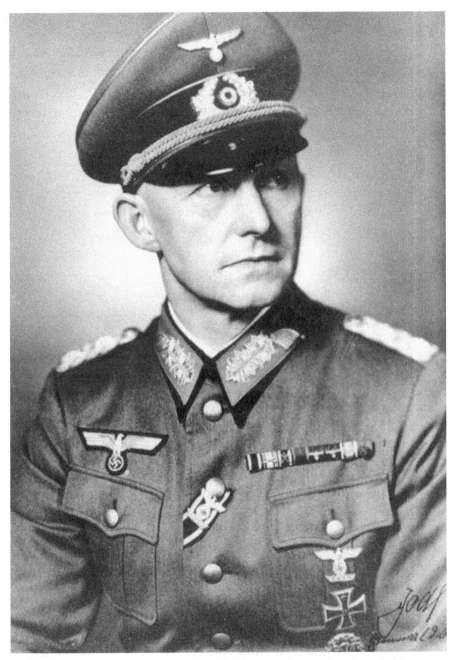

Alfred Jodl, Chief of Field Operations, who differed with Hitler regarding the goal of Operation Barbarossa. He argued for capturing Moscow as an additional strategic goal, resulting in dispersing the German military force over too broad an area. (Bundesarchiv, Bild 146-1971-033-01)

Germany at that time simply lacked adequate military equipment and manpower to achieve success.

Keitel disagreed with Hitler strongly enough that the Field Marshal presented a handwritten memo to Hitler in which he argued against Hitler's plan for a "preventative war on Russia." These efforts to convince Hitler were ineffective and predictably drew his wrath. Keitel received the expected tirade when he criticized the grandiose narcissist.

His thorough and angry dressing-down by Hitler caused Keitel to become despondent. Keitel went so far as to offer his resignation and request an appointment to a frontline command. Hitler refused Keitel on both counts. Hitler's lifelong tendency to develop rages following perceived criticism is demonstrated once again by this interaction with Keitel.

A further controversy erupted during the planning stages of Operation Barbarossa when, according to Keitel's memoirs, Alfred Jodl who served as the Chief of Operations of the Armed Forces High Command (OKW) and Halder argued that capturing Moscow should be the goal of the operation. Hitler similarly disagreed with Jodl, as he had with Halder, and opined that the goal should be taking Leningrad and Kyiv along with the vital gas and oil production facilities. Then in a somewhat uncharacteristic and conciliatory fashion, Hitler compromised and allowed for the inclusion of the additional thrust toward Moscow but not in lieu of Hitler's plan to take Leningrad, Ukraine, and the oil fields.

According to Keitel, Hitler only tentatively went along with the army's plan to take Moscow and signaled a change in plans would occur once Operation Barbarossa was underway. This promised change in the plan did not occur because of Hitler's unavailability due to illness (to be discussed later). The adding of the Moscow objective to Operation Barbarossa greatly extended the length of the front and the complexity of the battle plan.

ASPECTS AND FURTHER LIMITATIONS OF OPERATION BARBAROSSA

Operation Barbarossa began on Sunday, June 22, 1941. It was the largest German offensive of World War II and involved about four million Axis personnel along an 1,800-mile front. The tactics of the Panzers and their cooperation with the other German forces had been well worked out and described by Gen. Heinz Guderian. The striking initial success of Operation Barbarossa, like preceding blitzkrieg operations, relates to these carefully worked out tactics. Guderian prophetically proposed: "If the tanks succeed, then victory follows. Whenever in future wars the battle is fought, armored troops will play the decisive role. It is sometimes tougher to fight my superiors than the French. There are no desperate situations, there are only desperate people."

Despite the existing nonaggression pact with Stalin's Soviet Union, this momentous war in the east commenced and the Germans made progress until 1943. It was then that the German forces at Stalingrad were surrounded and ran out of munitions. The city fell back to the Soviets. The German defeat in this horrific conflict proved a major turning point in World War II. Following Stalingrad, the Axis forces were compelled into a grudging retreat, one that traded territory for time.

Operation Barbarossa became a conflict of attrition and brutal annihilation. The German *Abwehr* (Germany's military intelligence) had severely underestimated the Soviet army reserves. The initial encirclement strategy of Operation Barbarossa called for massing the German forces and invading Ukraine, cutting off the supply of food to Russia, and capturing not only the vital oil fields in the Caucasus but also the land bridge between the rivers Don and Volga (according to George Friedman's 2017 editorial in *Mauldin Economics*). By massing the German troops, encirclement of whole Russian armies was envisioned. The two additional prongs (attacking both Leningrad (now St. Petersburg) and Moscow) overextended the available German forces.

Due to the underestimation and fierce resistance of the Soviet forces, Keitel soon felt the German manpower requirements surge. Replacements were impossible to find. The Waffen SS siphoned off the cream of the crop according to Keitel, such that the army suffered both numerically in recruits as well as qualitatively. The fighting ability of the German troops also diminished the longer the campaign lasted due to loss of its bravest and best young officers.

Resupply became a major problem for the German troops. While the Nazis had earlier made the trains run on time, this proved impossible during Operation Barbarossa. The German railway transport system never met the needs of the German troops during Operation Barbarossa despite vast sums having been spent earlier on improvements in infrastructure. The scorched earth policy of the Soviets and the ripping up of the Soviet rail system along with destruction of the Soviet locomotives impaired German progress. Keitel reported that during the winter of 1941–1942 the performance of the railways turned disastrous. The existing trains simply could not supply the amount of matériel, provisions, and supplies required for the huge number of German troops.

Again, the question must be asked, had Hitler delayed the launching of Operation Barbarossa, would the outcome have been different? For example, beginning the conflict three to four years later when the broad-gauge mega-trains

(*Breitspurbahn*) were slated could have helped with their resupply difficulties at least up to the point where the tracks entered Soviet-dominated territory. The enhanced resupply would have increased the fighting capability of the German troops.

A second generally accepted strategic mistake for the Germans was coming as conquerors rather than liberators. Many Ukrainians sought separation from the Soviet Union and initially welcomed the Germans as liberators. But rather than treating the population as potential allies, the Nazis sought to annihilate them and create space for a growing German population. This second strategic mistake sprang from Hitler's and the Nazi Party's anti-Semitism and belief that the Slavs and Jews were inferior and had to be cleared from Ukraine or effectively made into slaves.

According to Walter Gorlitz in his 2000 book *The Memoirs of Field Marshal Wilhelm Keitel*, Stephen Fritz, and multiple other sources, Hitler on March 30, 1941, told the assembled 250 high-ranking German officers that the fight with the Soviet Union would be a fight to the death between two diametrically different political systems. As such, Hitler described how the war must be conducted without regard for the laws and customs of warfare. This urging by Hitler to ignore established and accepted military doctrine animated the annihilation of the conquered people.

LEBENSRAUM

Later in the summer and fall of 1941, Hitler issued his *Nacht und Nebel* (cover of darkness, or literally "night and fog") orders. The first directive held that German soldiers could not be held legally responsible for any untoward acts against civilians in the occupied territories. This removed legal ramifications from the slaughter of civilians by German military personnel.

The second directive permitted the killing of Red Army political commissars and the scorched earth policy. Hitler believed the scorched earth policy was necessary to drive the people from their farms and towns and to make room for Germany's expansion (*Lebensraum*). While the exact number of deaths of Soviet citizens (both military and civilians) during World War II remains contested, twenty-seven million losses has been generally accepted by Russia and the former Soviet Union.

Keitel claimed that his office accessed reports of degenerate warfare carried out by Soviet forces, and the various German directives were designed to emulate the dastardly actions of its enemy. However, his argument summoned little sympathy when he appeared before the Nuremberg Tribunal.

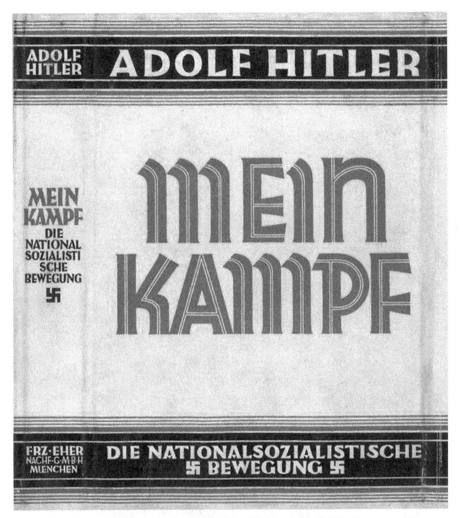

Dust jacket of *Mein Kampf*, in which Hitler argued for *Lebensraum* for the German civilization to survive and thrive. (Alamy stock photo)

As an aside, Field Marshal Keitel signed both orders on behalf of Hitler and by so doing signed his own death sentence. The Nuremberg Tribunal charged him as a "major war criminal." He immediately recognized that he would be found guilty including charges of waging a war of aggression; conspiracy to wage a war of aggression; violations of the laws or customs of war including murder, extermination, enslavement, and other inhumane acts against civilian populations. Keitel proved correct in his prediction and was found guilty at Nuremberg and hanged on October 16, 1946.

It was during the Barbarossa campaign that Germany had its greatest loss of life and weaponry during World War II. It was largely in Russia, Ukraine, and

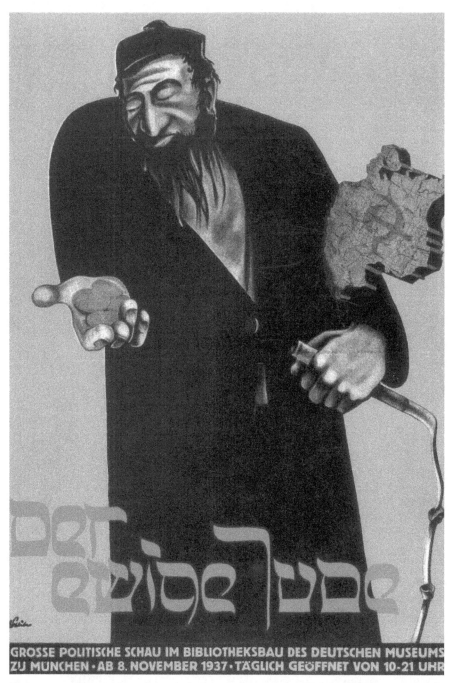

Nazi propaganda poster intended to depict Jews in the worst possible light. (Alamy stock photo)

Poland where the *Einsatzgruppen,* paramilitary German death squads, carried out their determined policy of extinction of Jews, political prisoners, Gypsies, and Slavic people along with a ruthless Germanization of the occupied territories. On September 28 and 29 alone, *Einsatzgruppen* massacred approximately 34,000 Jews at Babi Yar outside Kyiv. These atrocities served Hitler's fiercely held goal of achieving *Lebensraum*.

In a sense, the enlivening impulse of Operation Barbarossa derived from Hitler's *Mein Kampf*, written almost twenty years earlier. In his memoir that was more of a political manifesto, Hitler claimed Germans required more living space—*Lebensraum*. The expansive concept of living space had been around since at least 1901 when the geographer Friedrich Ratzel published an essay suggesting all civilizations needed to either expand their living space or else perish.

Whereas the French and British had established colonies around the world to fulfill their expanding demands for natural resources and trade, Hitler determined the German nation would be better served by seizing the land and resources to its east. Vast agricultural areas existed there along with vital oil reserves in the Caucasus. When appropriated by Germany, the results of the conquest would support Germany's growing economy and its envisaged manifest destiny.

Another book, published in 1926 by Hans Grimm entitled *Volk Ohne Raum* (*A People Without Space*), became a German classic and popularized Nazi Germany's belief for needing more living space. This book established the foundation for Hitler's *Lebensraum* by galvanizing the German people for what the war-weary German populace came eventually to view as a necessary war. Hitler believed such a war crucial and couched his argument in effective propaganda to capture the will of the German people. His dual purposes continued to be the eradication of both communism and Judaism.

Hitler regularly invoked racist rants against Jews, Slavs, and Gypsies to popularize the general acceptance of *Lebensraum*. Since the leaders of the Russian Revolution in 1918 and some serving in the Soviet government in the 1940s were Jewish, Hitler claimed Germany was fully justified in seizing their territory and resources. Hitler's prejudice and contempt were so all-embracing that he believed Slavs incapable of even ruling themselves, explaining why Jews had played such a key role in governing Russia. Although Hitler held great contempt for Jews, he held their administrative abilities in higher regard than those of Slavs. Hitler's hatred of Jews and other "inferior races" seemingly knew no bounds.

Hitler predicted in *Mein Kampf* that exterminating the Jews would cause the fall of the Soviet Union and wrote:

It [the prior Germanic governing class of Russia] has been replaced by the Jew. Impossible as it is for the Russian by himself to shake off the yoke of the Jew by his own resources, it is equally impossible for the Jew to maintain the mighty empire forever. He himself is no element of organization, but a ferment of decomposition. . . . And the end of Jewish rule in Russia will also be the end of Russia as a state.

Anti-Slavism was a principal component of Nazism and was reinforced by Hitler's many public rants. The Nazis believed that Slavs were a subhuman race and the citizens of the Slavic countries, principally Poland, Serbia, and Russia, could never be considered part of the Aryan race.

Hitler held out some hope for a small portion of the non-Jewish population in Slavic countries who could trace their origins back to a Germanic lineage. These ethnic Germans might be spared, if willing to be "Germanized." This exception was especially true for blue-eyed, blonde-haired women in the conquered territories who would participate in the *Lebensborn* program where they would become impregnated by members of Hitler's SS. The resulting *Lebensborn* children were then taken from their mothers and sent back to Germany where faithful supporters of Hitler could raise them as Nazified Germans.

Hitler's construct of *Lebensraum* became Germany's policy during the Third Reich. This belief sprang in part from misinterpreted anthropology ostensibly bolstering the Nazi claim that Aryans had once ruled the world. The Nazis claimed Cro-Magnon man originated in Germany and that this species had emptied Europe of less advanced Neanderthals. This incorrect portrayal of anthropology provided the Nazis a historical parallel for twentieth century extermination of "inferior" Slav and Jewish people. This superior minded and racist attitude of the Nazis also mistakenly led to the underestimation of the military prowess of Slavic countries, especially Russia—a fatal flaw in Hitler's dreams for conquest.

Hitler had hoped the 1936 Olympics would tout the superiority of Aryan athletes over the inferior races of the world. Germany did succeed in leading the overall medal count with a total of eighty-nine medals, a remarkable feat considering its medal count four years earlier had been only fifteen at the Los Angeles Summer Olympic games. While Goebbels attributed this improvement to Aryan superiority, it is known that German Olympic athletes in 1936 used amphetamine injections to enhance their athletic performances. Had this pharmacological aspect been widely known, it would have diminished Hitler's argument for Aryan genetic superiority. Nevertheless, an African American named Jesse Owens reduced Hitler's festive attitude by winning four gold medals in high-profile track events at the 1936 Olympic games.

As an aside, one cannot help but wonder what Hitler and the Nazis would have thought of our modern understanding of the human genome. Whereas the Germans, Jews, Russians, Poles, Italians, English, and all other European peoples are known to possess a small percentage of the Neanderthal genome (the complete set of DNA in a Neanderthal), Hitler's argument of Aryan supremacy and annihilation of the Neanderthals fails completely. Moreover, the African races viewed by Hitler and the Nazis as inferior are the only populations in Europe and Asia not possessing Neanderthal genes.

While the policy of *Lebensraum* makes the argument for more space for an expanding pan-German population, *Lebensraum* in no way explains Hitler's haste to invade the Soviet Union in the early summer of 1941. The next chapter will present health-related information that further elucidates Hitler's timing for the invasion of the Soviet Union.

BEHAVIORAL AND MEDICAL INFLUENCES ON OPERATION BARBAROSSA

MEGALOMANIA AND MENTAL INFLEXIBILITY

Hitler's megalomania reduced the chances of success for Germany's invasion of the Soviet Union. In his 1970 memoir *Inside the Third Reich*, Albert Speer, the Nazi Minister of Armaments from 1942 to 1945, recounted his recommendation given in July 1941 that all building operations not in service to Operation Barbarossa or the overall war effort be suspended. A disagreement broke out between Speer and a Dr. Fritz Todt from the building industry. Speer eventually won Todt over to his argument, only to have Hitler overrule his plan for military prioritization. While Speer's plan would have increased the likelihood of Barbarossa's success, Hitler's megalomaniacal desire for immediately remaking Germany into an architectural wonder and world capital overrode Speer's prudent planning.

Even Speer, the architect of the planned ambitious building campaign, did not believe other projects, even his own, were so important for Germany as to starve the overall war effort of necessary supplies. Hitler could simply not bring himself to halt his favorite building projects, e.g., the autobahn, Party buildings, and various Berlin and Nuremberg projects, despite their competition for valuable war-necessary materials and funding.

In his memoir, Speer derisively described the awarding of thirty million much-needed Reichsmarks to leading stone companies in Norway, Finland, Italy, Belgium, Sweden, and the Netherlands for the purchase of granite for grandiose Berlin and Nuremberg building projects. Speer knew that existing German resources were inadequate to tackle these public endeavors and simultaneously build up the necessary armaments needed for military success.

Even during the winter of 1942 when the military operations in Russia were not proceeding according to plan, Speer quotes Hitler as saying, "The building must begin even while this war is still going on. I am not going to let the war keep me from accomplishing my plans."

Hitler envisioned a broad new avenue in Berlin where a huge domed meeting hall would be built, so large that all of St. Peter's Cathedral in Rome could have been easily placed within it. To match this massive construction, on the other side of the avenue Hitler planned a colossal Arch of Triumph that would rise four hundred feet into the air. He thought this structure would be a worthy monument to the German war dead. Such was Hitler's detachment from reality, resulting from his megalomania and grandiose narcissism.

Hitler also began to demonstrate mental rigidity and difficulty in changing his mind despite the introduction of new information and clear-cut limitations. Such inflexibility in thinking were consistent with his neuropsychological findings associated with his advancing Parkinson's disease.

STUBBORNNESS AND SCAPEGOATING

A second feature of Hitler's abnormal personality, his profound stubbornness and inability to recognize his errors, also diminished success in Operation Barbarossa. Wilhelm Keitel, head of the German High Command, in his memoir stated, "Early in 1941 the drive for Tikhvin in the north, which the *Führer* had tactically launched against the War Office's advice, suffered a reverse." The commander, a field marshal, asked for freedom to reposition his troops and permission to withdraw from part of his front. Hitler denied permission and instead demanded the commander's resignation. Keitel thought Hitler sacrificed two first-class commanders during this episode, only to provide scapegoats for setbacks that resulted from his own unwillingness to acknowledge his blame.

ACUTE ILLNESSES INTERVENE

Dysentery also intruded on Hitler's conduct of the war in the east. This acute illness occurred not long after Hitler's argument with Joachim von Ribbentrop in July 1941. Hitler fell ill with a severe bout of dysentery, incapacitating him for several vital weeks. During this time, Hitler's generals managed to scrap his encirclement strategy and mounted the additional full-frontal assault on Moscow (the German Army's preferred plan).

Recall that Hitler had earlier indicated he would cancel the Moscow attack once the campaign was underway. According to David Stahel in his 2009 book *Operation Barbarossa and Germany's Defeat in the East*, Hitler and Halder, head of Army General Staff, fundamentally disagreed on how the operation should be conducted and the intermediate objectives. Earlier in the planning this disagreement had gone unsettled. Hitler's acute illnesses during August and September 1941 provided Halder and the Army General Staff leeway to conduct the attack on Moscow.

In his weakened state, Hitler proved unable to fight for his original encirclement plan. Hitler had envisioned massing German troops, encircling large numbers of Soviet troops, and starving the Soviet Union of its food and fuel. He saw the taking of Moscow, the Soviet capital, as unnecessary.

Hitler's illnesses undercut his effectiveness during the heaviest fighting on the Eastern Front. While under interrogation after the war, Hermann Göring posited that had Hitler's original encirclement strategy been maintained, Operation Barbarossa would have succeeded, and Germany would have conquered the Soviet Union. Field Marshal Wilhelm Keitel held the same opinion.

The precise cause of Hitler's dysentery during the first half of August 1941 remains unknown but the duration and severity suggest bacterial dysentery, such as salmonellosis, shigellosis, or staphylococcal food poisoning. Hitler's illness lasted three vital weeks. These first two varieties are worldwide and result from poor sanitation. Both begin with colicky abdominal pain and fever. The lack of pathological bacteria from Hitler's stool sample argues against these two bacterial varieties according to Professor Alfred Nissle who did the laboratory examination.

Staphylococcal food poisoning is a third variety and may be the most likely form of acute gastroenteritis to have struck Hitler. The duration of the dysentery, however, is long for staphylococcal food poisoning unless he repeatedly ingested contaminated food.

Certain strains of staphylococci produce an enterotoxin. This form of enteritis usually results from foods contaminated by food handlers who have superficial infections or provide nasal droplets containing staphylococci. Poor refrigeration frequently gives rise to this disorder. Cream-filled pastries, custards, and sweets of the type Hitler loved to consume are common sources of the staphylococcal infection.

Symptoms of staphylococcal food poisoning usually begin within six hours following ingestion of the bacterial enterotoxin. The onset is abrupt with severe nausea, vomiting, and cramping abdominal pain. The illness is prostrating. Indeed, Morell chronicled that Hitler was forced to go to bed. A person with dysentery feels quite ill, and Hitler in this case would not have been capable of carrying out critical thinking regarding an invasion of the Soviet Union or arguing over possible alteration of tactical or strategic matters.

The cause of the staphylococcal enteritis could only be determined by analysis of the foods that were contaminated. The course of the illness generally runs to under a week. In Hitler's case, given his lifelong irritable bowel symptoms, the symptoms of gastrointestinal upset, and possible continued ingestion of contaminated food, the duration might have lasted longer.

At the time of Hitler's dysentery, he stayed at the Wolf's Lair in eastern Prussia. This sprawling but primitive headquarters lay in swampy land within a forested area. Hitler had joked that the land must have been very inexpensive or else already have been public land because he could not imagine any other reason why it would have been purchased. Mosquitoes made residing at Wolf's Lair unpleasant along with the added discomfort of living in a damp, cold bunker. Such an environment as Wolf's Lair is a far cry from the tropical climates where dysentery more often occurs. Nevertheless, a lack of proper sanitation or refrigeration as noted above can cause dysentery and likely existed within the bunker at Wolf's Lair.

Dr. Morell worried that Hitler might have contracted a bacterial or parasitic form of dysentery. The fecal samples Morell sent to the medical lab revealed none of the bacterial or parasitic causes for dysentery known at the time but did not exclude campylobacter (a common foodborne illness from eating contaminated food or drinking contaminated water that can lead to an infection of the gall bladder) or to viral causes of dysentery or a pathogenic variety of *E. coli*. Such variants of *E. coli* were not understood at the time to cause dysentery.

Morell apparently became sufficiently nervous over the *Führer*'s acute illness that on August 7, 1941, he began writing regular clinical notes in Hitler's casebook. Soon afterward Morell began two days of treatment with Yatron, a medicine for amebic dysentery. Morell must have believed, due to the limited sanitation in the Wolf's Lair bunker, that amebic dysentery was a likely diagnosis. He also treated Hitler with various multivitamin preparations. The test results of Hitler's stool that Morell had sent earlier to Freiburg returned on August 5. Professor Alfred Nissle, the discoverer of Mutaflor, reported that the sample contained no infectious germs or parasitic worm eggs.

Since amebic dysentery is diagnosed by identifying under the microscope the Entamoeba histolytica, the tiny disease-causing agent—an examination that Professor Nissle performed—it is unlikely that Hitler had amebiasis. The fact that Professor Nissle gave Morell a negative report on August 5, and Morell began treatment for amebic dysentery on August 9, is difficult to reconcile. Dr. Morell proved once again that he was a therapeutic enthusiast of the first order.

Perhaps Morell feared missing a serious cause of dysentery that carried the possibility of widespread abscesses. After all, Morell had an existing therapy for amebic dysentery, whereas he did not have effective antibiotics for salmonella or shigella-induced dysentery, or for the various viral causes. Also, Morell may once again have simply fallen prey to his well-known penchant for overtreatment and a desire to be viewed by Hitler as "doing something."

In late September shortly after his prolonged bout of dysentery, Hitler fell ill from yet another gastrointestinal disorder. At that time his second gastrointestinal illness caused jaundice as mentioned in an earlier chapter. His eyes became distinctly yellow. Hitler suffered severe colicky abdominal pain, nausea, and reported that his urine had turned "brown as beer." Morell examined Hitler's belly and found it taut and tender. Morell treated him with a synthetic morphine product for the pain and a spasmolytic medicine to relax the contractions of the intestinal tract.

Hitler's symptoms as described by Dr. Morell suggest a gall bladder attack. I recall a lecture in medical school where the professor of medicine described the experience of suffering such an attack as a "profound sensation of utter doom." After having personally experienced such an attack, I hold the opinion that my medical school professor underestimated the patient's utter misery during such an attack.

It can be safely said that Hitler would not have been able to defend his preferred aggressive military plan during such a debilitating illness. Again, this second gastrointestinal illness, presumably a gall bladder attack, came at a most inconvenient time, occurring during the heaviest fighting and when Hitler was most needed to frustrate the General Staff's planned assault on Moscow.

This presumed gall bladder disease led to "the doctor conspiracy" and discussion of jaundice along with other general health matters. To briefly reiterate, Dr. Hans Karl von Hasselbach and Dr. Karl Brandt believed Morell's use of Dr. Koester's anti-gas pills with their small amounts of strychnine were causing Hitler's jaundice. Morell strongly disagreed that this consideration was even a possibility, and initially went further by denying Hitler had jaundice at all. A spirited medical disagreement occurred among Hitler's cadre of doctors that led to Hitler firing both von Hasselbach and Brandt.

As an aside, in addition to being Hitler's personal surgeon, Brandt also achieved notoriety in another way. He directed and participated in the infamous medical experiments at the concentration camps and directed the euthanasia projects. For these crimes against humanity Brandt was later tried by the Nuremberg courts, condemned to death, and executed in 1947.

In retrospect this bout of abdominal discomfort with jaundice was likely a gall bladder attack, coinciding with what Morell had assumed at the time. His impression of a gallstone blocking the common bile duct would explain Hitler's attacks of abdominal pain, jaundice, and flatulence.

The final arbiter of this diagnostic dilemma should have been the autopsy performed on Hitler's partially burned body by the Soviet forensic pathologists in 1945. This report will be more fully covered in a later chapter. Suffice it to say, the politically influenced autopsy report, while listing spurious, politically motivated findings, fails to even mention Hitler's gall bladder.

Hitler's gastrointestinal issues caused discomfort severe enough to incapacitate him for weeks at a time. While not having the overall strategic impact of Hitler's neurological and cardiac illnesses, these gastrointestinal disorders rendered Hitler ineffective at a historically critical time. Undoubtedly the lack of a healthy Hitler impaired the effectiveness of Operation Barbarossa by allowing the army to carry out the added objective (the capture of Moscow, the Soviet capital), thereby diluting the effectiveness of the invading German forces.

CHAPTER 18

DR. THEODOR MORELL

Any discussion of Adolf Hitler's health would be incomplete without further mention of Hitler's controversial private physician, Dr. Theodor Morell. To understand the strangeness of Hitler's health care, it is important to understand the relationship that existed between a controlling and noncompliant patient and an anxious-to-please and avaricious physician.

THE MYSTERIOUS ALLURE OF THEODOR MORELL

Who was this doctor in whom Hitler bestowed such confidence and what role did Morell play in assisting Hitler, so that *der Führer* could continue with his exhaustive, high-level work?

Morris Leikind in his declassified US intelligence report written in 1945 held that Hitler liked quacks. Hitler was said to like astrology, the study of sleep walking, and magic. Among the tenets of the Nazi Party could be found antivivisectionists, disbelief in vaccinations, and strong believers in vegetarianism. Fringe elements of science held allure for Nazis. Dr. Morell fit right in with those who held these strange beliefs.

BRIEF BIOGRAPHY OF HITLER'S PERSONAL DOCTOR

Dr. Theodor Morell was born in Upper Hesse on July 22, 1886. He served as a medical officer during World War I. Reminiscing about their common experiences in World War I and their shared disappointment over its outcome undoubtedly surfaced in idle conversation between these two disgruntled World War I veterans. Morell joined the Nazi Party early in 1933, and as mentioned earlier, came to Hitler's attention when Hitler's friend and photographer Heinrich Hoffmann required treatment for a venereal disease.

As a general doctor with special interest (but little training) in venereal diseases and skin disorders, Morell knew little about neurology, cardiology, or gastroenterology—areas of expertise that better coincided with Hitler's nervous system, heart, and gastrointestinal illnesses. Despite his lack of medical sophistication and his virtual shunning by Hitler's better-trained and respected physicians, general practitioner Morell enjoyed Hitler's absolute trust. Up to very near the end of Hitler's life, Hitler believed him to be nothing short of a medical genius.

David Irving's book *The Secret Diaries of Hitler's Doctor* chronicles Morell's medical journals of Adolf Hitler. Following World War II, these medical records were lost until March 1981 when Robert Wolfe, a US Army officer and senior archivist of the US National Archives, received a telephone call from the Department of Health, Education and Welfare, stating the Morell files had been discovered.

Review of Morell's journals in Irving's book shows how the doctor was quick to deviate from the standard medical practice of the day, flattering Hitler by telling him that his importance to Germany required accepting inherent risks of using incompletely proven, as well as anecdotal, therapies. Others in Hitler's employ referred to Morell's methods in more negative terms, such as frank quackery. Such a radical approach as Morell used might well have appealed to Hitler given the Nazis' ready acceptance of fringe science. The Nazis also showed an overt suspicion of academia with its dull and established ways, favoring more extreme approaches, often based on little more than inference.

Leonard and Renate Heston in *The Medical Casebook of Adolf Hitler* theorize Morell treated Hitler with methamphetamine and that the treatment eased Hitler's fatigue. As discussed previously, Dr. Karl Brandt became suspicious of Hitler's dramatic resurrections following an injection from Morell and had Hitler's medicine identified. Brandt determined that Morell was indeed administering methamphetamine.

The Hestons in their work *Adolf Hitler: A Medical Descent That Changed History* also suggest that Hitler developed a dependence on methamphetamine. Although aware of the threat of methamphetamine complications, Morell nevertheless chose to keep "Patient A" pleased with his care and administered "what he needed." An established dependence on methamphetamine further secured Hitler's attachment and need for his controversial and unconventional general doctor.

PATIENT HITLER

Adolf Hitler must have been any doctor's worst nightmare. As any doctor knows, one of the most difficult patients to manage is one who self-diagnoses and demands specific and frequently incorrect treatments. *Der Führer* was just

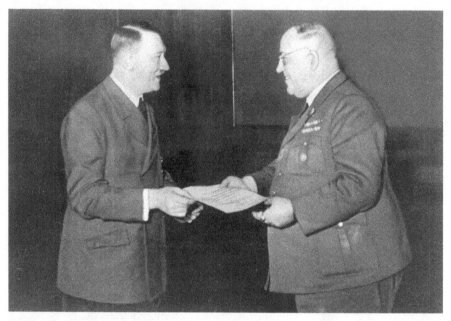

Dr. Theodor Morell (right), Hitler's controversial personal physician. (Alamy stock photo; Süddendeutsch Zietung Photo, Alamy, Image ID: C45C58)

this type of patient. In his blustery, haranguing way, Hitler would tell Morell what treatment he needed, while refusing either physical examination or medical investigation. For example, when having abdominal colic, Hitler would demand Eukodal, a synthetic morphine (strongly constipating and habit forming), and Eupaverin, a strong spasmolytic. Morell would dutifully inject Hitler with those agents, although not standard therapy, and the two medicines worked at odds to each other. The combination of a controlling patient and a compliant, anxious-to-please physician made for a dangerous situation and poor medical care.

Hitler insisted Morell treat his symptoms, while refusing diagnostic examinations such as chest X-rays or increased frequency of his electrocardiograms, due in part, Hitler claimed, to great demands on his time. Both Hitler's stubbornness over providing sufficient time for diagnostic studies and excessive modesty prevented Morell from examining parts of Hitler's body. Even though Morell held himself out as expert in urology, no record exists that he ever examined Hitler's genitalia (other than performing cremasteric reflexes) or that he ever performed a rectal examination.

To test for cremasteric reflexes the doctor lightly strokes the inner thigh with a needle to observe the intact reflex: elevation of the testicle on that side. One can imagine Hitler holding a towel over his penis to preserve his modesty, or else

Morell peeking up Hitler's ballooned German underwear (fashionable in the day) to observe whether the testicle retracted upward.

Given the extent of Hitler's bowel complaints, the lack of performing a rectal exam shows extraordinary negligence. In instances where Hitler required an enema, Morell would sit dutifully outside the bathroom door, listening attentively, hoping to hear telltale sounds of Hitler's constipation breaking up and bowel gas escaping.

The ever anxious-to-please Morell was quick to comply with Hitler's wishes, and in so doing prescribed dozens of different oral medicines as well as injections. The latter approach he was particularly keen about, often giving 10 to 20 percent glucose solution and Vitamultin (an ineffective vitamin preparation) injections several times a day. Hitler's intake of medicines included several painkillers, stimulants, sedatives, laxatives, sleeping pills, cardiac tonics, medicines to improve digestion, pick-me-ups to increase manliness and sexual performance, along with various vitamin and hormone preparations.

LATE CARE PROVIDED BY MORELL

According to Morris Leikind, Morell's administration of medicines in the latter stage of his employment was almost entirely by injection. This change in route of administration was likely added for its showiness rather than any added medical benefit.

Morell began providing preventative treatments as well. He gave injections of a sulfa drug—manufactured by his own factory—not only to Hitler but also to those around him. He assumed that the sulfa antibiotic would ward off colds and flu. Of course, this antibacterial treatment provided no benefits whatsoever for viral colds and flu and merely left Hitler and his associates with sore rumps. When Hitler felt symptoms of a cold coming on, Morell would provide him with six to eight painful injections of sulfa daily. In retrospect perhaps it is not surprising that Hitler stood throughout many of his briefings. Morell would also provide prophylactic injections the day prior to a scheduled Hitler speech when the forecast predicted inclement weather.

Morell appears not to have shared his knowledge of Hitler's high blood pressure and coronary artery disease with Hitler's other doctors. Likewise, Dr. Erwin Giesing, an ENT doctor who disliked Morell, did not communicate information regarding his own treatment of Hitler with cocaine. Different physicians not communicating their treatments, then as now, may give rise to dangerous polypharmacy with risks for medicine interactions and duplication.

During the spring of 1945 and the terminal phases of World War II, Hitler became extremely distressed and paranoid over what he imagined were attempts to drug him and physically remove him from Berlin. His regular use of methamphetamine may have brought on this paranoia. The methamphetamine, along with exhaustion, fear, and depression regarding the long course of the unsuccessful war, contributed to Hitler's distrustful state of mind.

In this state, Hitler ultimately became convinced that Morell was part of a plot to drug and then spirit him out of Berlin. As a result, Hitler summarily fired Morell on April 21, 1945. Morell does not elaborate in Hitler's casebook on this momentous action beyond providing the date and terse entry, "dismissed!"

While Morell had loyally descended the stairs into the *Führerbunker* with Hitler, no doubt fully expecting to die there with him, Morell's unexpected dismissal probably saved his life. Once discharged from Hitler's service, Morell left the bunker and managed to escape Berlin on one of the last German flights out of the city. Before making his breakout, he left behind a large amount of prepared medicine for Hitler to be administered by another of Hitler's doctors or Hitler's valet.

During these desperate days at the end of the war, Morell's thoughts must have returned to what he believed had been earlier commitments from a grateful Hitler. Without Morell, Hitler had believed that he would not live long enough to pursue his plans for a Greater Germany. Morell must have recalled Hitler's promise that if they successfully conducted World War II, then he would be richly rewarded. Had the war turned out differently Hitler would likely would have lavished additional riches and prestige on his loyal personal physician.

Leikind described that under Hitler's patronage Morell had built factories and manufactured patent medicines. In some instances, Morell had secured favorable purchase arrangements with the government including compulsory purchase of his medicines for all German citizens. In other instances, Morell was granted a monopoly for his brands of medicine. Hitler's patronage had made Morell wealthy and successful, at least for a time.

In May 1945 the American military captured Morell—a man by then reduced in body, wealth, and spirit. He was incarcerated and interrogated.

MORELL'S FAILING HEALTH AND DEATH

By the time of his escape from Berlin, Morell's own health had deteriorated, as he suffered from kidney disease and cardiac insufficiency. When Morell had sent Hitler's electrocardiograms to Dr. Arthur Weber, he also sent along his own electrocardiograms. Morell's heart tracings showed even more prominent and advanced disease characteristics than did Hitler's tracings.

After the fall of the Third Reich and while in custody, Morell developed such poor health that he could not be properly interrogated. He had by then suffered a stroke that impaired his ability to speak. One of his American interrogators shared his disgust over Morell's lack of hygiene and gross obesity. Attempts were made to interrogate him at an American internment camp at the site of the Buchenwald concentration camp. Morell's debriefing proved largely unsuccessful, and he was never charged with a crime.

As Theodor Morell lay with his right arm and leg paralyzed and unable to express his thoughts verbally, one wonders what thoughts occupied his mind. Had Nazi Germany won World War II, Morell might have gained his own institute, enjoyed great wealth, and been widely respected. He could have bought all the fineries his wife desired and splurged on fine foods and beverages. Instead, at the end of his life Morell lay in a shabby hospital, wearing a diaper, and possessed a clouded mind. His reputation along with his health had been thoroughly shattered.

Morell died May 26, 1948, in Tegernsee, Germany. He died a broken, confused, and impoverished man. His wife Hannelore Moller Morell died the same year. The cause of death as listed on Theodor Morell's death certificate was stroke.

CHAPTER 19

RISING DEMANDS AND INCREASED MEDICATIONS

Both coronary artery disease and Parkinson's disease are slowly progressive disorders. While the war dragged on, factors internal to Adolf Hitler inexorably diminished his physical and mental abilities to perform his increasingly demanding political and military tasks.

PROGRESSION OF HITLER'S ILLNESSES

While hastening Operation Barbarossa may have reduced its chances for success, the struggle along the Eastern Front still lasted for almost four years. The available medical records are limited and fail to reflect milestones documenting Hitler's disease progression. This blank in medical records of "Patient A" from September 1941 to July 22, 1942, leaves a huge gap.

We can assume that along with his untreated moderate high blood pressure that the atherosclerosis in Hitler's coronary arteries also slowly progressed. Without angiography or other imaging techniques of his coronary arteries—procedures that did not exist at the time—the progression would have been impossible to document except by the worsening of Hitler's clinical symptoms.

Likewise, his Parkinson's disease can be assumed to have progressively slowed his movements, stiffened his muscles, diminished his facial expression, reduced his articulation, and increased his hand tremor. Of these features, Morell documented only Hitler's tremor as substantially increasing. In each instance Morell interpreted an increase and an extension of Hitler's tremor to heightened stress levels and increased fatigue associated with the various battles being fought. Of course, acute stress or anxiety does transiently increase tremor, but Morell failed to recognize his underlying and advancing neurological disease.

Morell ascribed Hitler's slowing of movements, mentation, and other symptoms to depression (so-called psychomotor retardation of depression). Admittedly, the diagnosis of depression can be challenging in a Parkinson's disease patient, as the usual reduction of physical activity and mental slowing of clinical depression are also features of Parkinson's disease.

When assessing for depression in a patient with Parkinson's disease, specific questions need be asked to tease out feelings of worthlessness, sadness, and dysphoria (a generalized feeling of ill-being) that indicate the presence of clinical depression. Morell failed to carry out any such mental status assessment. That is not to say that reactive depression did not exist in Hitler, especially during times where the German forces encountered military reversals, only that Dr. Morell may have lacked the clinical sophistication to tease out what portion of psychomotor retardation was due to unrecognized advancing Parkinson's disease, and what part resulted from reactive clinical depression. Lack of effective pharmacological therapy for both entities at the time makes this point largely moot, although some psychiatric support might have been offered to Hitler.

During the remainder of 1942, Hitler's health records also reveal substantial intestinal problems with excessive gas and constipation along with complaints of headaches. Several mentions of a swollen and tender temporal artery are included in his medical records. This finding suggests temporal arteritis and could explain his complaints of serious headache.

Temporal arteritis (better known as giant cell arteritis) is a medical disorder in which an inflamed artery, frequently but not always the temporal artery that runs along the side of the head, becomes swollen and extremely painful. This disorder occurs usually in people beyond the age of fifty who are of northern European descent, as was Hitler. The cause is unknown but thought to relate to the body's autoimmune response. It can give rise to fatigue, loss of appetite, and serious visual symptoms that may include sudden visual loss. A biopsy of the affected artery demonstrating the pathological findings of giant cell arteritis might have confirmed the diagnosis in Hitler. Adolf Hitler never had a biopsy of his painful artery, and current treatment with steroid medications was, in any event, unavailable in Hitler's day. As such we can neither confirm nor deny that temporal arteritis in Hitler was present.

AN ATTRIBUTIVE CONTROVERSY ARISES AGAIN

A popular 2017 book titled *Blitzed* by Norman Ohler focused entirely and in detail on the impact of drugs on Hitler and the war. This book again drew attention to the outsized role of narcotics, cocaine, and methamphetamine usage within the Third Reich. Ohler is a journalist who spent years researching the widespread use of such pharmaceuticals within the German military and among its citizens.

This book awakened the old disagreement described earlier in the preface, as Volker Ullrich panned the volume as sensationalist and claimed that it sought to revive the old idea that Morell had gotten Hitler hooked on drugs. Ullrich, like some other writers, seemed distrustful of medical influences on Hitler and argued the drugs prescribed for Hitler had less to do with his physical deterioration than did his permanent overexertion and unhealthy lifestyle. He particularly thought Hitler needed more physical exercise.

Earlier in this book the work of Leonard Heston was presented along with his assertion that Hitler received regular methamphetamine treatments with dramatic results. No doubt, this treatment with its habit-forming tendencies and serious side effects had negative impacts on Hitler, as did the chronic exhaustion claimed for Hitler by Ullrich.

These various factors, be they historical or medical/psychological, combined to bring about Hitler's deterioration. All the factors deserve consideration and authors can disagree on their order of impact. While Ohler's book may be sensationalist, it clearly points out the overuse of narcotic, stimulant, and other habit-forming agents by Hitler.

It is assumed that Ullrich recoiled from Ohler's book due to concern that Hitler might be forgiven for having been addicted to medications. Such an excuse might be viewed by some belated fans of Hitler as offering mitigation for his horrendous crimes. As we shall see, such concerns for relieving Hitler of his overwhelming guilt seem greatly exaggerated.

USE OF NARCOTICS

Dr. Morell treated Hitler's complaints of severe headache in 1943 with injections of Eukodal. Today this is better recognized as oxycodone or by its brand name, OxyContin® (an extended-release preparation). Other brand names of oxycodone include Percocet® and Percodan®. This medicine had been around since 1917 and according to Norman Ohler was deemed in Hitler's time the "queen of remedies." It was twice as strong a pain reliever as morphine and extremely popular then (and now with its illicit usage). Its popularity grew because Eukodal

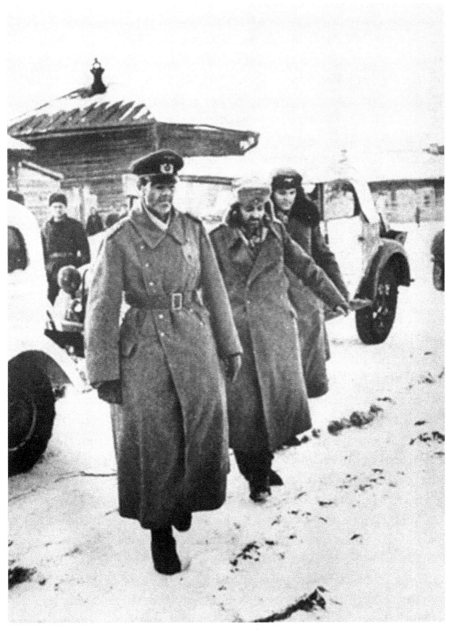

Gen. Friedrich Paulus, surrendering to the Soviets at the Battle of Stalingrad. Despite being elevated by Hitler to the rank of Field Marshal, Paulus refused to kill himself for "that little corporal." (Alamy stock photo; Image ID: EK3FNE/ ITAR-TASS News Agency)

(oxycodone) is known to give rise to a rapid euphoric state even greater than that caused by heroin.

Because of its strong addictive tendency, Morell worried about using the drug. Regular usage of Eukodal (oxycodone) can cause dependency in as little as three weeks. He nevertheless relented and administered Eukodal just prior to an important meeting that Hitler had with Benito Mussolini. He gave Eukodal to Hitler by subcutaneous injection. None around Hitler could have failed to notice the striking increase in his energy level and improved temperament following the injection.

While the treatment was risky, Morell deemed the danger acceptable in view of the catastrophe for the Axis alliance should Hitler not be available to meet with the leader of the second largest Axis power. Hitler liked the sensation provided by Eukodal so well that he wangled a second injection prior to Mussolini's departure, this time receiving the injection intramuscularly.

Indeed, Hitler greatly appreciated his Eukodal therapy with its attendant psychological effects and thanked Morell frequently for what he viewed as his highly beneficial treatments. Once exposed to the Eukodal, Hitler would not relinquish it. As we now know, oxycodone is strongly addicting, a fact that in fairness to Morell was not as well appreciated in the 1940s. Morell, nevertheless, tried to use Eukodal only on alternate days, to reduce Hitler's chances for addiction.

WORSENING OF MILITARY SITUATION ON THE EASTERN FRONT

Military reversals in North Africa and Stalingrad in late 1942 and early 1943 increased Hitler's workload and heightened his anxiety. A request from Gen. Friedrich Paulus to surrender at Stalingrad in late January met with Hitler's resolute refusal and an emotional outburst. Instead of agreeing to Paulus's request, Hitler decided to promote Paulus to the rank of Field Marshal.

Hitler knew that no German Field Marshal had ever surrendered. By promoting Paulus Hitler attempted to lock Paulus into the distressing position of either continuing to fight or committing suicide. Despite his promotion to Field Marshal, Paulus surrendered his defeated Sixth Army to the Soviets. Paulus commented disparagingly that he saw no reason to die for that "little corporal."

Throughout this stressful period Morell injected Hitler at regular intervals with glucose and a variety of tonics. To this witch's brew came the introduction of still another habit-forming agent—cocaine. The introduction of cocaine occurred at perhaps the most stressful period for Hitler since he was gassed in World War I.

OXYCODONE AND COCAINE

Several weeks following the Allies' successful landing on the beaches of Normandy and the establishment of a second front, Col. Claus von Stauffenberg and other frustrated confederates tried to assassinate Hitler at Wolf's Lair in eastern Prussia. The operation known as Operation Valkyrie attempted to take over the government. The failed Operation Valkyrie inadvertently led to still greater pharmacological consequences, again nicely described by Norman Ohler in his 2017 book *Blitzed.*

In addition to his cuts and splinters, Hitler's eardrums were blown out, leading to blood seeping from both ear canals. Morell heard the explosion and headed for Hitler to render service as quickly as his rotund body would allow.

Soon thereafter Morell injected Hitler with substance "x." The nature of this injection remains open to question but likely was the narcotic Eukodal. This treatment enlivened Hitler, allowing hundreds if not thousands of splinters to be removed from his legs. It also vastly improved his mood but did nothing for his bleeding eardrums or his temporary loss of hearing.

Dr. Erwin Giesing, an ear, nose, and throat specialist from a nearby field hospital, was summoned to deal with Hitler's bleeding ears. Dr. Giesing found his patient pale, with a swollen face and bloodshot eyes. Hitler's speech was unnaturally loud, due to his recent loss of hearing. He also appeared aged and physically depleted according to Dr. Giesing.

To treat the pain in Hitler's ears, Giesing used cocaine drops, not knowing that Morell had already injected him with a narcotic. Cocaine, a powerful local anesthetic, provided additional pain relief for Hitler. The variety of cocaine administered was a potent 10 percent cocaine solution that would have given rise to a strong euphoria in Hitler. It was not long before the addictive personality of Adolf Hitler began seeking additional cocaine, and he became demanding for more. While Giesing tried to maintain his medical scruples to a greater extent than did Morell, he eventually gave in to Hitler's demands and prescribed cocaine at frequent intervals.

The cocaine along with the opiates and methamphetamine provided Hitler a pleasing pharmacologically altered reality despite the worsening of the war. Hitler's staff during this period frequently commented on his good moods and budding confidence, leading them to believe that surely Hitler must have had some grand plan up the sleeve of his military tunic that would rescue Germany from a looming defeat. Little did they know that Hitler was responding, as do most users of these addictive substances, by exhibiting a drug-induced euphoria.

CHAPTER 20

IMPACT OF HITLER'S PARKINSON'S DISEASE ON THE BATTLE OF NORMANDY

H itler's chronic Parkinson's disease altered his cognitive function, and the cognitive/memory losses affected his performance as a military leader, particularly evident around the time of the Battle of Normandy.

BACKGROUND TO THE BATTLE OF NORMANDY

The second front, long demanded by Joseph Stalin, began in June 1944. While Winston Churchill had promoted a second front elsewhere "in the soft underbelly" of Europe, both the United States and the Soviet Union favored an invasion of northwestern Europe. According to historian Volker Ullrich, Hitler knew that the outcome of an invasion in the west would determine the outcome of the war.

The buildup of Allied forces in England was well known to Germany. Surprisingly, Hitler was excited by the possibility, believing an invasion repulsed would provide time for his military to refocus on the Eastern Front. According to Stephen Fritz, Hitler considered the Allied invasion a great opportunity and that the planning for such a vast undertaking was complex. If the Allies failed, it would take them at least another year to mount a second invasion. Such a victory by the German forces might convince the Allies that they could not win the war, would deal a blow to Churchill's political position, and might even cost President Franklin Roosevelt reelection in the United States.

The question as to where and when the invasion would occur, however, was uncertain. The two most likely options according to German thinking consisted of the narrowest part of the English Channel at the Pas de Calais or, as a second viable alternative, the Normandy coastline and Cotentin Peninsula. To address Hitler's Atlantic Wall, Field Marshal Erwin Rommel was tasked with reinforcing the coastline. Hitler was pleased with Rommel's increased fortifications and happy that he had put the final touches on them. Hitler invited the Allies to try their luck against this military barrier and by so doing smash themselves to smithereens.

Likewise, Rommel was optimistic according to Ullrich's writing: "In the west, we are quite confident of getting the job done." He also wrote his wife in mid-May 1944 and mere weeks before the invasion, "We get stronger day by day." Rommel also was pleased by the praise Hitler lavished upon him for his good work in preparing the Axis defenses. Later historians with the benefit of hindsight have questioned the German optimism given that the Allies had overwhelming naval and air support. In addition, the German defensive fortifications had weak points and many of the Axis forces were not the crack units that had largely been deployed to the Eastern Front but instead included many non-German Axis forces (see Fritz, Ullrich, Kershaw).

One major reason for Germany's inability to fend off the Allied invasion related to its slowness to respond. Therein Hitler's physical and mental health played a role in working against the Axis forces.

THE DITHERING NAZI

The loss of Hitler's mental flexibility that led to difficulty in his handling contradictory reports impacted the outcome of the Battle of Normandy (also referred to as Operation Overlord or D-Day). Hitler's initial response (or lack thereof) at this battle proved to be one of the most decisive errors of World War II.

The historian Stephen Ambrose in his 1995 writing *D-Day: What Went Wrong* listed three major reasons why the Germans lost at Normandy. First, the Allied attack at Normandy proved a complete surprise to the Germans due to the bad weather and lack of a well-organized, timely counterattack. Second, confusion on the part of the Germans was rampant due to a lack of air reconnaissance (the Allies had near complete air supremacy), telephone lines blown by airborne troops and French partisans, and initially the absence from Normandy of commander Field Marshal Erwin Rommel. Third, the German command structure proved an utter disaster because of Hitler's constraints on the distribution of the German divisions.

According to Ambrose, the only high command German officer who responded correctly at the outset of this battle was Field Marshal Gerd von Rundstedt. Nevertheless, Hitler had earlier removed Rundstedt's authority to position division strength troops, such that Rundstedt at the onset of the battle proved to be little more than gray-clothed window dressing.

When three divisions of Allied paratroopers (two American and one British) began parachuting behind the Normandy beaches in the early hours of June 6, Rundstedt recognized the airborne attack for what it was—the prologue to an invasion force. While his messages back to Hitler kept open the option that this assault could be a feint, he believed strongly that this was the beginning of the real invasion.

Rundstedt soon concluded that such a show of force from the Allies inevitably must be followed by an invasion, and that this airborne attack was certainly not a military feint. He understood this assault to be the major attack from the Allies and that they intended to establish Normandy as the Western Front. Quite correctly two hours before the seaborne landings began, Rundstedt ordered two reserve Panzer divisions (the Twelfth SS Panzer and the Panzer Lehr) to counterattack at Normandy. While Rundstedt's reasoning proved sound, his actions decisive, and his orders clear, the Panzers were no longer under his control. Instead, Hitler had earlier assumed command regarding the distribution of all German divisions, and the two Panzer divisions failed to move under what would have been the cover of darkness and heavy skies.

While not involved in the military decision-making, Albert Speer happened at the time to be at the Berghof with Hitler when the Battle of Normandy began. He recounted his observations about that day in his memoir *Inside the Third Reich*:

> . . . at the Berghof around ten o'clock in the morning when one of Hitler's military adjutants told me that the invasion had begun early that morning.
>
> "Has the Führer been awakened?" I asked.
>
> He shook his head. "No, he receives the news after he has eaten his breakfast."
>
> In recent days Hitler had kept on saying that the enemy would probably begin with a feigned attack to draw our troops away from the ultimate invasion site. So, no one wanted to awaken Hitler and be ranted at for having judged the situation wrongly.

Orders prior to Hitler's awakening then came from the Chief of Operations of the German General Staff Alfred Jodl to Field Marshal Rundstedt. Jodl ordered that the two Panzer divisions in question could not be committed until Hitler gave his approval. On learning of Jodl's order, Rundstedt rescinded his earlier, all-too-prophetic order to counterattack immediately. Instead of mounting a Panzer attack toward the beaches of Normandy that General Rommel had previously identified as the likely invasion site, the two German Panzer units halted and awaited orders from a sleeping Hitler.

It is of interest according to Stephen Fritz that Rommel's experience in Italy favored locating all the Panzer divisions closer to the coast, as the Allied air power had previously exacted heavy losses prior to the Panzers' joining the battle. Rundstedt on the other hand preferred that the Panzer divisions be located some distance away in a central area. This massing of force was Wehrmacht doctrine and was supported by Gen. Leo Geyr von Schweppenburg, the commander of Panzer Group West. From such a more distant vantage point the Panzers would be able to strike in force at their target once the invasion site was clearly identified. It was believed by the German planners that the German naval and air forces could greatly damage the invading armada and that, should the Allied forces come ashore, they could then be demolished by the later arriving Panzer divisions.

To settle the strong disagreement between Rundstedt and Rommel, Hitler divided the tank forces with two divisions tied down at the Pas de Calais and the remaining divisions grouped closer to Paris. This decision by Hitler in retrospect proved a worse strategy than would have either strategy proposed by Rommel or Rundstedt. This "Panzer controversy" according to Fritz would end up exposing the lack of clear lines of authority in the German military.

According to Churchill, still further confusion was sown by 14,600 Allied sorties compared to a mere one hundred German sorties flying over Normandy during the early stages of the battle. A lack of German heavy bombers reduced the capacity to defeat the invading armada and beachheads. The Allies held overwhelming air superiority and carried out extensive bombing and strafing raids. These raids inserted confusion, diminished Nazi communications, and inflicted substantial losses among the German defenders.

German Luftwaffe leadership had earlier considered building heavy bombers but rejected this step because during the Spanish Civil War the two-engine bombers had proved more accurate. Much of the Luftwaffe's failure to defeat England in the Battle of Britain sprang from its lack of just such long-range bombers that could savage England's industry and military buildup.

Likewise, the Allied naval vessels scored successes. On learning of the large invasion armada moving toward the shores of France, a stream of German U-boats

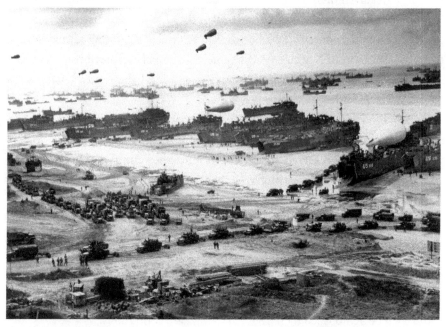

Photo of D-Day landing at the Battle of Normandy, showing extensive invasion forces. (Alamy stock photo)

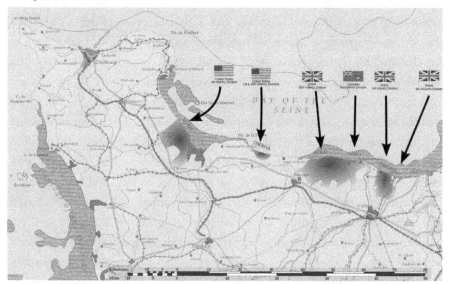

Map of the Allies' approach for the landing forces on the beaches of Normandy. (Operations Greenwood and Pomegranate Normandy July 1944 EN.svg: Philg88 Derivative work: Hogweard - Operations Greenwood and Pomegranate Normandy July 1944 EN.svg CC BY 4.0)

departed at high speed from the Biscay ports to intercept the Allied invasion armada. The western approaches to the channel proved well guarded by the Allies, and the U-boats fared badly in the exchange of fire. As such, the U-boats had little to no effect on the Allied invasion.

Along with the aerial bombardment, shelling from offshore Allied battleships and cruisers poured down upon the German positions, stunning the German defenders. The combination of Allied bombing and shelling suppressed German fire until the landing forces came within a mile or so of the beaches. The bombardment also largely interrupted German radar, further limiting accurate firing from the German big guns.

The weather proved a factor and further worked against the German defenders. During the morning of June 6, a heavy overcast hung like a gray pall over the Normandy beaches. This heavy weather would have protected the two Panzer divisions from aerial attacks had they been released. Around 4 p.m. Hitler finally gave his approval of a very limited counterattack the following morning, but by then the skies had cleared and the Panzer divisions became exposed to withering air attacks. The Panzers sustained heavy losses.

The heavy seas from the storm the day before caused the German command to believe the invasion was impossible. Field Marshal Rommel became so convinced of this weather-related invasion delay that he had left his post at the Normandy front to attend his wife Lucie's forty-seventh birthday party that happened to fall on June 6. When the Battle of Normandy began, Rommel was far away from Normandy and settling in for a festive birthday celebration.

At 6:30 in the morning on June 6, 1944, Allied troops began storming ashore at the Normandy beaches. Imagine the alarm of the German defenders when dawn broke, and they gazed out from their defensive positions in stark amazement and morbid fascination at the huge armada splayed out in front of them. On spotting the Allied armada and suffering the impact of the bombing and artillery campaign, the shaken German defenders immediately recognized the huge scale of the assault and called for reinforcements. No doubt the German defenders hoped for the release of the two Panzer units and the Fifteenth Army reserves that were located near and around the Pas de Calais.

The urgent request of the German defenders at Normandy was very slow to reach Hitler. Hitler slept and slept, and upon waking at noon, dallied over his breakfast. Hitler may have suffered the type of sleep disorder previously discussed with Parkinson's disease consisting of insomnia, excessive daytime sleepiness, and slowness to arouse.

It is well known that Hitler had a habit of staying awake until the wee hours of the morning while engaging in conversation, and then not waking until late in the morning or midday. Hitler's sleep pattern proved true to form the night before the Battle of Normandy in that he had stayed up until 3 a.m. and then slept to midday. His somnolence and dithering likely associated with his Parkinson's related sleep disorder may have proved costly to the German cause. A changed strategy became necessary to defend against the invading forces; however, no order for reinforcements was forthcoming. Hitler's lack of leadership at this juncture and coordination of the German military response reduced the chance for a German victory at Normandy.

Hitler's well-known emotional rages also likely benefitted the attacking Allies at Normandy. Despite alarming reports streaming in from Normandy, none of Hitler's staff would dare to wake him, fearing that if they did, they would be targeted by his fury. When Hitler finally awoke and learned of the requests for release of the Panzers and other reserves, he categorically denied them. Hitler believed the real invasion would come at the Pas de Calais and that the Normandy incursion was the expected Allied tactical feint.

ALLIED DECEPTIONS

Hitler's incorrect presumptions had been carefully cultivated through Allied misinformation. Allied deceptions had fostered dissention and confusion between Hitler and some in his High Command regarding the site and timing for the invasion of France. This propaganda and misinformation campaign by the Allies had been designed specifically for this purpose and succeeded in thinning the German ranks at Normandy.

As the American, British, and Canadian troops prepared for their invasion of France, they also carried out extensive operations to deceive the German High Command as to the location of the invasion, all of which is nicely described in Winston Churchill's 1953 book *Triumph and Tragedy*. One of these deceptive efforts involved Gen. George Patton whom the German High Command held in high esteem and who was the general they assumed would lead the Allied invasion of France.

A counterfeit army was built around Patton that included inflatable phony trucks and tanks. The location of Patton's phantom army lay directly across the English Channel from the Pas de Calais region, providing presumptive evidence for Calais as the invasion site. This location of Patton's faux army represented the shortest distance between England and France, making it the logical site from which to launch the invasion. From Patton's supposed encampment emanated deceptive radio transmissions that added to the Allies' ruse.

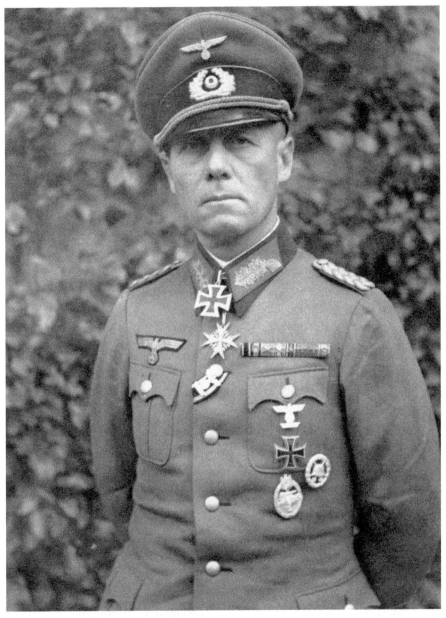

Gen. Erwin Rommel, who correctly identified the vulnerability of the German forces at Normandy and sought to improve the German defenses. He championed meeting any invasion on the beaches. (Bundesarchiv Bild 183-J16362)

Other false reports were fed to the Nazis via double agents in England, suggesting still other sites for the Allied invasion. This false information helped to disperse the sixty German divisions over a wide area of France and even Norway rather than concentrating their forces in a militarily sound way at the Allies' chosen invasion site. The Allied deceptions slowly firmed up the belief in Hitler and his generals that the invasion would most likely occur at Calais or possibly another site and not at Normandy. It is of interest that Hitler earlier believed that Normandy was the likely site of the invasion, adding further support to the effectiveness of the Allied misinformation campaign.

Rommel disagreed with the German Command's assumption and correctly surmised the attack would come at Normandy. Given the increasing centralization of the military decision-making that had been firmly placed in Hitler's hands, Rommel's opinion regarding the Allied invasion site proved of little or no benefit for the German defenses.

On the second day of the Battle of Normandy, the Allies solidified their shaky beachheads, of which Omaha Beach was in the greatest jeopardy. While the German defenders mounted a counterattack—Hitler relented slightly by releasing one Panzer unit that attacked on June 7—the vital Fifteenth Army reserves and the other available Panzer divisions played no part in it (Churchill, *Triumph and Tragedy*). The limited First German Panzer counterattack failed to turn back the invading forces. According to Churchill, so convinced was the German High Command and Hitler of a second full-scale attack that the reserves of the Fifteenth Army remained south of the Pas de Calais a full six weeks following the initial invasion of Normandy.

The correct site of the attack at Normandy soon became apparent to Hitler's commanders; however, this determination made little difference in Hitler's thinking. Hitler clung tenaciously to his incorrect conviction regarding the site of the Allied invasion. He continued to believe for far too long that the Allied attack was a mere feint.

IMPACT OF PARKINSON'S RELATED MENTAL INFLEXIBILITY AND PERSONALITY

Hitler, due to his Parkinson's related mental inflexibility, lifelong stubbornness, and inability to admit his own mistakes, simply could not readily give up his false belief. He held onto his false beliefs beyond the time that a normal person would require to change his or her mind to fit with evolving circumstances.

Adolf Hitler was fifty-five years old, had suffered from Parkinson's disease for more than a decade, and proved unable to assimilate the overwhelming evidence streaming into his headquarters. Within this emotional caldera of conflicting reports and amid the fog of war, Hitler must have felt overwhelmed and confused as to what was truly unfolding in the north of France. His mental inflexibility, even obstinacy, prevented a timely alteration in the German military plans that doomed the German defense to fail.

It should be reaffirmed that Hitler had the final say in the disposition of all German divisions. He ignored the demands of Field Marshal Rundstedt, the commander in chief of the Western theater of war, to centralize the Panzer divisions and the opinions of Field Marshal Erwin Rommel who had been charged with defending France and who wished to have the Panzer divisions close to the beaches. The compromise satisfied neither commander. The centralized reserve units had been held back specifically by Hitler's order, failing to utilize the night of June 6–7 to move the German units forward. This delay allowed the Allied bombers to inflict heavy losses on the reserve Axis troops and equipment, even prior to encountering the Allied ground forces.

On June 8, two full days after the invasion began, Hitler reluctantly released additional military assets from the already battered German reserves. By then the Allies had dug in, off-loaded armor and additional combat and logistical troops, and were able to repel this delayed German counterattack. The German armored counterattack proved too little and too late.

The presence of the Normandy front meant Germany then had two fronts to defend, overstretching the Axis's military might beyond its capabilities. The German loss of the Battle of Normandy and the establishment of a second front predetermined the outcome of World War II.

Winston Churchill's work *Triumph and Tragedy* attributed Hitler's slowness to respond at Normandy solely to carefully orchestrated Allied deceptions. No doubt intelligence misinformation including Patton's phantom army strategically placed across the English Channel from Calais proved important, but it may not entirely explain the German military's delay in counterattacking.

In addition to these intelligence deceptions, the neurological explanation helps to explain Hitler's dithering that resulted from his mental inflexibility, difficulty in shifting his thoughts based on new information, and diminished executive function due to his chronic Parkinson's disease. Simply put, Adolf Hitler could not rid himself of his previously held notion as to where the attack would come. His slowness to respond was reflected in his indecisive leadership. Hitler's cognitive dysfunction was also abetted by his lifelong stubbornness and slowness to accept criticism or admit his errors. These factors created the perfect mental storm that mirrored several days earlier the stormy weather in the English Channel.

Further examples exist of Hitler's failure to heed the advice of his top military commanders throughout the remainder of World War II and to respond in a timely fashion. Hitler continued to throw tantrums, dress down associates, and replace high-ranking officers for failing to follow his increasingly impractical orders. He was unwilling to accept information that ran counter to his previous and stubbornly held notions.

Tragically for loss of life and property, Hitler steadfastly persisted with the war despite Germany's then near hopeless military situation. Germany's ultimate futility resulted from degradation of its troop strength, armaments industries, and fuel storage capacity and led to Germany's total defeat in World War II.

GERMAN MILITARY FRUSTRATIONS BOIL OVER

On June 20, 1944, Col. Claus von Stauffenberg and other co-conspirators made their unsuccessful attempt to assassinate Hitler. The coup d'état leaders sought to form a German government acceptable to the Western Allies in the hope of establishing a truce, thus preventing their homeland from being overrun by the Soviets. Hitler's inability to accept this grim reality, despite its obviousness, doomed Germany to total defeat and destruction. The von Stauffenberg assassination plot stemmed from growing frustration from some in the German military and arose from Hitler's overbearing conduct of the war and his failure to follow the advice of his commanders *in a timely way.*

CHAPTER 21

BATTLE OF THE BULGE

Five months after the Allies' successful invasion at Normandy, Hitler launched his riskiest assault in one final attempt to turn back the encroaching Allies. The combination of his heart disease, neurological disease, and strange assortment of medicines further hindered his ability to act as the decisive, insightful leader that was greatly needed at the time by Nazi Germany.

A RISKY MILITARY GAMBLE REFLECTING HITLER'S MENTAL STATE

The last great World War II battle on the Western Front began December 16, 1944, and ended on January 25, 1945 (History.com, *The Battle of the Bulge,* October 14, 2017). The careful planning of the German offensive had taken much time. Hitler personally had spent months poring over maps, engaging in planning sessions with top staff, and developing the invasion plan for the Ardennes. He had considered various counteroffensives that might alter the Axis powers' slow arc toward defeat. He also increasingly spent time quarrelling with generals whom he viewed as timid and who persisted in offering multiple but less ambitious plans than those favored by Hitler.

Speer in his book *Inside the Third Reich* recounted that following the Battle at Normandy and when the German military situation began seriously to deteriorate, Hitler began to dismiss the advice of others:

> Hitler closed his mind more to any word against his decisions. He proved to be more autocratic than ever in this action. This hardening of his mental arteries had crucial consequences in the technical area as well; because of it the more valuable of our "secret weapons" were made worthless [reference to the ME- 262 jet fighter].

Hitler's all-in, risky plan for his surprise counteroffensive in the Ardennes never gained more than grudging support among his top generals. Hitler, who was supremely confident in his judgment and as stubborn as always, nevertheless bulled ahead and implemented his plan. Clearly the disparity between the Allied and Axis forces at this stage of the conflict predicted Germany would lose the war.

Hitler's hope was that if he could split British forces from the American forces, then he could effectively force Britain out of the war. As he viewed the situation, such a military reversal would cause the United States to reconsider its enthusiasm for the war and negotiate a peace treaty. Hitler in effect had little to lose at this point, as the war was going decidedly against Germany. This risky venture for Hitler seemed worth the gamble, given his fierce determination to establish Germany as a great power and his unwillingness to surrender.

Importantly, Hitler also demanded that not a single detail of his plan be altered, effectively handcuffing his generals from making necessary tactical changes during the inevitable unpredictability of the battle. Despite the limited fuel and waist-deep snow, Hitler ordered his top commanders Walther Model and Gerd von Rundstedt along with Gen. Sepp Dietrich to follow his orders precisely, orders that included Hitler's immutable directive "not to be altered."

Hitler repeatedly recalled with gleeful pride the first Ardennes battle fought August 21–23, 1914, in World War I in which the German armies soundly defeated the French forces. Hitler's recollection of this favorable turn of events contributed to his confidence in his plans for the Battle of the Ardennes in the Second World War.

THE BATTLE BEGINS

The morning of December 16, 1944, broke cold with a leaden sky hovering like a pall over the Ardennes Forest (located in Belgium, Luxembourg, and northern France) where the great battle would unfold. The bad weather initially grounded all Allied aircraft including its observation planes. The heavy skies benefitted German operations by masking their advancing forces and preventing the Allies from utilizing their substantial air superiority in fighters and bombers.

For Hitler this battle represented a final, high-stakes throw of the dice, as he knew that for the war to continue along the same downward path Germany would inevitably lose. The Axis forces launched Hitler's huge offensive referred to as Operation Watch on the Rhine (*Unternehmen Wacht am Rhein*). Later in the battle, due to stretching (or bulging) of the Allied lines and thanks to vivid newspaper accounts in the West, the battle would become better known as the Battle of the Bulge.

The German name for the operation sprang from a German patriotic song. In the event of an intelligence leak, it was thought, the name of the offensive would construe a limited defensive operation, rather than the huge offensive attack that it truly represented. The plan had been designed to split apart the armies of the Western Allies. Specifically, it was intended to cut off the British and Canadian armed forces in the north from the American forces in the south, retake Antwerp, the major seaport for the Allies, and create enough consternation and pain among the Western Allies to enable Germany to force a separate truce. If successful, the operation would remove the major Western Allies from the war and allow the German forces to redirect their remaining military strength against the Soviet Red Army.

It was truly a desperate gamble by Hitler. Fortunately for the Germans, it also played well into the prevailing sense of overconfidence among the Allies, who acted as if the war was virtually over. Secrecy about the battle plan was crucial for Germany's success. By both limiting those who knew about the assault and restricting the amount of German radio traffic, Hitler managed to keep his ambitious invasion plans secret.

The entire powerful Axis force of close to a million men and 1,400 tanks extended along an eleven-hundred-mile front, but the breakthrough was designed to take place in the American Ardennes sector. To gather such firepower from the already depleted German military proved a huge logistical effort. The Germans had to remove many of the battle-hardened troops and armor from the Eastern Front and, without being detected, transfer them to the Western battle lines.

The initial surprise German attack consisted of 200,000 troops and 350 to 400 tanks and mobile artillery pieces that had been amassed along the American lines in the Ardennes. The attack began at 5:30 a.m. with 1,500 big guns heralding the offensive with a ninety-minute barrage. The artillery spat fire and steel and wreaked havoc among the stunned American troops, as they frantically tried to dig foxholes in the snowy Ardennes Forest using their hands, helmets, and bayonets. The German attack killed and wounded many troops, considerably thinning the American lines.

Hitler had selected the Ardennes Forest due to the ruggedness of the terrain and forested landscape. These features made the site an unexpected place to launch such a major attack. Indeed, this sector was known among the Western Allies as a quiet one where nothing much ever happened, and where new troops could be sent for training and more experienced troops assigned for rest and relaxation.

The German offensive called for a lightning attack led by Hitler's favorite tank ace, Joachim Peiper. A vital key for success was tremendous operational speed,

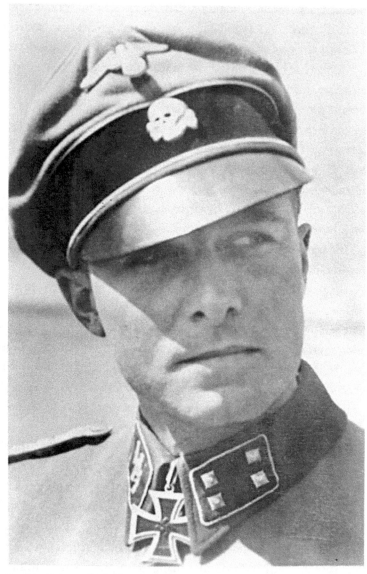

Joachim Peiper, a field officer in the Waffen-SS who was Hitler's favorite tank commander. He led the German attack at what became known as the Battle of the Bulge. (Bundesarchiv Bild 183-R65485/ CC-BY-SA 3.0)

speed sufficient to capture intact bridges over the river Meuse and the much coveted and needed fuel dumps. Hitler demanded maximal speed be taken as fuel and munitions would not last long enough for a slow, slogging assault.

By late 1944 fuel for the German Army was in critically short supply, and the Germans lacked sufficient reserves of fuel to move their attacking troops all the way to Antwerp. Capturing the Allies' fuel dumps became an imperative if the operation was to prove successful. This assumption of capturing fuel depots intact was risky at the outset and proved to be so in actuality.

The strategy within the more limited German Operation Greif, as it was called, was to utilize English-speaking German commandos, dressed in American uniforms, and led by Otto Skorzeny who would precede the advancing Panzer armies. Their mission was to sow chaos in the Allied troops' rear by interrupting communications, issuing fake orders, and seizing key strategic points. Their efforts caused paranoia among the American troops, giving rise to checkpoints being thrown up where questions thought only Americans could answer were asked of unrecognized individuals. Such questions included naming state capitals, sports questions about baseball team affiliation, and trivia questions about American culture.

This improvised tactic even snared English Gen. Bernard Montgomery who had the tires of his vehicle shot out and was for a time detained in a barn until his identity could be confirmed. American Gen. Omar Bradley also had to prove his identity and answer questions about Betty Grable and football before being allowed to pass a sentry point.

Operation Greif proved largely unsuccessful, as the German airdrop was not well executed and scattered the commandos. This poor implementation resulted in many commandos being captured and some being shot as spies. The German commandos also suffered from too few competent English speakers, too few American uniforms, and only limited knowledge of "Americanisms" to successfully succeed in the face of the impromptu questioning.

The two main German military forces to exploit the bulge in the Allied line were the Fifth Panzer Army led by Hasso von Manteuffel, recipient of the Knight's Cross, and the Sixth SS Panzer Army led by Josef "Sepp" Dietrich. Hitler had handpicked these two trusted generals. Both Manteuffel and Dietrich were loyal Nazis. Sepp Dietrich had even at one time served as Adolf Hitler's chauffeur and bodyguard prior to 1929. It was in performing this task that Dietrich had first won Hitler's trust.

The resistance offered by the inexperienced American troops shocked the German military leaders. Nowhere was this resistance more prominent and heroic than in the defense of the small town of Bastogne, a location from which many critical roads fanned out. The limited number of men defending Bastogne proudly referred to themselves as "the Battling Bastards of Bastogne." This small village proved a critical way station for the German Panzer armies. It needed to be taken quickly and passed through hurriedly during the Panzers' sprint to the river Meuse. From there the Panzers would speed on to the deep-water port of Antwerp.

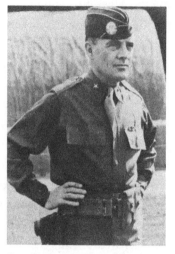

Gen. Anthony McAuliffe, acting
commander of the heroic US 101st
Airborne Division at Bastogne.
(US National Archives)

The American 101st Airborne stationed near Bastogne had different ideas. At the outset of the operation these American forces rushed into Bastogne and held off a much larger and better equipped German force just long enough to allow Patton's Fourth Armored Division to disengage, pivot ninety degrees, and arrive in Bastogne on December 26.

Many people today are familiar with the now famous American response from Bastogne to the Germans' demand for surrender. The pithy response by the acting commander of the Bastogne forces, Brig. Gen. Anthony McAuliffe, simply read, "Nuts, from the American Commander." Initially the meaning of the cryptic American response baffled the German major receiving the message. When he asked Col. Joseph Harper who had delivered the American message what the response meant, Colonel Harper, knowing that General McAuliffe avoided profanity, interpreted the message in more typical army-speak by saying, "It means Go to Hell!"

As early as December 18 (two days after the battle began), Hitler's point man Field Officer Joachim Peiper had already bogged down and had become frustrated by his lack of rapid progress. While his start had been successful and had surprised the Americans, Peiper soon found himself getting further and further behind schedule. Several times, because of roadblocks and blown bridges, Peiper had to change the direction of his tanks. Peiper also learned that American troops fought far more tenaciously than expected and that they gave ground only reluctantly.

GERMAN OFFENSIVE GRINDS TO A HALT

Stiff resistance at the villages of Malmedy and Stavelot slowed Peiper's progress even more. The German force at Malmedy captured and then massacred eighty-four American prisoners of war. The American prisoners had been held in a field where they were machine-gunned rather than taken to a prisoner of war camp. A few escaped the massacre and spread the word as to what had happened, further hardening American resistance. For these heinous actions Peiper became forever known as the Butcher of Malmedy. His desperation to claim the American fuel dumps that were necessary to reach Antwerp along with Hitler's firm insistence on rapid progress resulted in Peiper taking these drastic and inhumane actions.

Peiper and his Panzers eventually arrived at Trois Ponts, presenting him at last with a welcome tactical opportunity. He knew that if he could cross the Amblève River by way of the town's three main bridges, good road lay ahead. This passage would allow his tanks to dash through the Belgian countryside and reach the river Meuse in mere hours.

As Peiper's lead tanks ground up the road and approached the bridges, American tanks swung into position. An engagement ensued but had barely begun when tremendous demolition blasts occurred that destroyed the vital, timesaving bridges. To his horror, Peiper saw the bridges explode and tumble down into the river Amblève. He sat in his tank, thunderstruck, staring at the airy expanses that then existed where minutes before the bridges had firmly stood.

The thwarted German commander was forced to move still further north to Cheneux. Peiper's forces arrived after a long and disappointing day. Again, just as his tanks moved within two hundred yards of his planned crossing over the river, the bridge over the Lienne River disappeared in a cloud of smoke and amid a deafening roar. The bridge collapsed into the river along with Peiper's final hopes for military success.

With the loss of this bridge Peiper's advance stalled. He radioed back to headquarters and asked for help. He soon learned a German relief column would not be coming to his rescue. The lack of further support placed him in an almost hopeless position. He was told in accord with Hitler's orders not to retreat. Again, Hitler's stubbornness, mental inflexibility, and grandiosity were evident that day.

Peiper's failure to achieve his mission resulted from the bravery of American engineers, tankers, sappers, and even rear-guard soldiers including truckers and cooks. By then Peiper was pressingly low on fuel, short on ammunition, and dreadfully behind schedule. He again signaled his superiors that he needed to retreat to save the lives of his men as he was out of fuel and ammunition. Hitler's

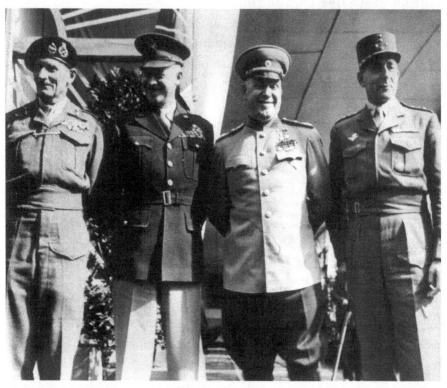

Allied forces commanders, Berlin, 1945. Left to right: Field Marshal Bernard Montgomery, Gen. Dwight Eisenhower, Gen. Georgy Zhukov, Gen. Jean de Lattre. (Alamy stock photo CW716T)

stubbornness was again displayed when he refused to accept Peiper's desperate plea. Hitler viewed Peiper's entreaty as defeatism. He again ordered Peiper not to retreat but rather to fight to the death.

IMPACT OF HITLER'S MENTAL RIGIDITY

Hitler was unable to rapidly process and accept Peiper's impossible situation. Hitler had foreseen a dramatic and rapid breakthrough of the American lines and simply could not quickly react to battlefield realities. Hitler's mental inflexibility due to his advanced Parkinson's disease and lifelong personality characteristics were again on full display. He was unable to process accurately the incoming intelligence and changes required by shifting battlefield conditions. He was besotted by the way the plan was supposed to work and unable to rapidly change his military responses based on current battlefield exigencies.

No doubt during this chaotic fog of war, Hitler believed his plans were not being carried out as intended. His lifelong suspiciousness fell upon his commanding officers, believing that they simply were not trying hard enough. Rapid changes in plans that were required simply could not be processed due to the mental inflexibility of Adolf Hitler.

The attack had not gone as planned and Peiper lacked the necessary fuel, ammunition, and firepower to pursue the attack further. Peiper's request had come, after all, from Hitler's favorite tank commander who in the past had shown great bravery and had won many prior battles. Ultimately Joachim Peiper had little choice but to ignore Hitler's direct order. He and his men abandoned and destroyed their tanks and fled on foot into the forest. They slowly picked their way back to the German lines. More than seven hundred of the original eight hundred men under his command eventually made their way back to the safety of the German lines.

The attack as planned by Hitler and his largely reluctant commanders had been brazen and overreaching. Some 20,000 American casualties occurred during the battle compared to 120,000 German casualties. In addition to the grievous and irreplaceable loss of manpower, Germany also lost huge numbers of tanks, half-tracks (vehicles with regular front wheels for steering and continuous tracks at the back to propel the vehicle and carry most of the load), artillery pieces, and precious remaining fuel reserves.

The intransigence blended into the offensive war plan reflected Hitler's mental inflexibility and his unwillingness to allow his troops to improvise according to battlefield conditions. These factors contributed to Germany's defeat at the Battle of the Bulge. The loss of this last great battle on the Western Front accelerated Germany's defeat in World War II.

Hitler's lifelong, egotistical stubbornness was on display during the Battle of the Bulge. Hitler's mental inflexibility and inability to readily incorporate new information, as seen with advanced Parkinson's disease, prevented Hitler's mind from readily accepting new and breaking information, and prevented a change to more effective tactics. Hitler could not even envision a way his army could lose this battle. He remained convinced that his Aryan troops were acclimated to harsh winter conditions and possessed better strategy and fighting ability than the perceived weaker men of the Allied armed forces. Hitler clearly showed overconfidence, mental inflexibility, grandiosity, and once again underestimated his enemy. These factors accrued to Hitler's defeat at the Battle of the Bulge.

The German loss at the Battle of the Bulge signaled to the Axis forces that the war was lost. It had been a final, desperate gamble to force a truce with the Western Allies and allow Germany to pit all its military forces against the invading Soviet forces. While Hitler tried to maintain morale among his underlings by

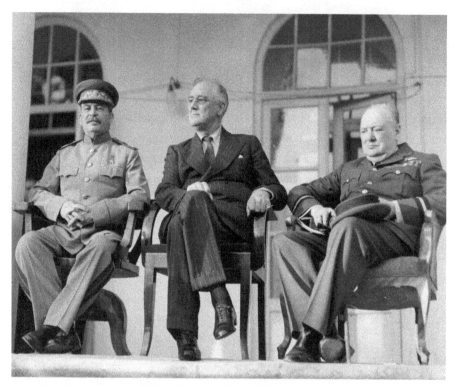

Soviet Premier Joseph Stalin, US President Franklin D. Roosevelt, and British Prime Minister Winston Churchill, meeting at the "Big Three" Tehran Conference in November–December 1943. (US National Archives 197062; Franklin D. Roosevelt Library, Public Domain Photographs 1882–1962)

making unrealistic predictions, he too could not have escaped knowing that the end of the war and his own leadership would soon arrive. He likely began considering his personal options including his ultimate escape, capture, or death. He was bound to have understood that his time as *Führer* of the Third Reich was increasingly limited.

CHAPTER 22

THE REMAINS— HITLER'S AUTOPSY

An autopsy represents the most complete physical examination a person will ever receive. As such it frequently answers lingering diagnostic questions and sometimes provides unexpected pathological findings. Given the importance of Adolf Hitler's medical diagnoses and their impact on the twentieth century, Hitler's autopsy should be of paramount importance and provide tantalizing conclusions regarding his health and his death. But, as suggested earlier, Hitler's autopsy fails to deliver the goods. Nevertheless, it is worth reviewing the saga that Hitler's autopsy represents as reported by Soviet forensic pathologists. The report shines light on attendant Soviet political issues and explains the sprouting of conspiracy theories ever since.

The most widely accepted story of Adolf Hitler's death is that he and his wife of less than two days, Eva Braun, committed suicide in the bunker on April 30, 1945. When the Soviet Red Army had reached within five hundred yards of overtaking their place of refuge, Eva Braun is believed to have taken her own life by biting down on a cyanide capsule. Hitler is believed to have died from a self-inflected gunshot to the head (and possibly from simultaneously biting down on a cyanide capsule).

Their dead bodies were then wrapped in a carpet by Hitler's staff, lugged up the stairs of the bunker by SS soldiers, and taken into a nearby garden where they were placed in a shallow depression caused by an exploding artillery shell. The two bodies were then drenched with gasoline and burned for several hours before being covered with dirt. While this scenario is the most widely held and corroborated by eyewitness accounts, conspiracy theories abound including the last-minute escape of Adolf and Eva from the bunker and ultimately from Germany. Conspiracy advocates have claimed that Hitler lived to a ripe old age in such faraway places as Argentina, Bolivia, Japan, and even the South Pole. These rumors of escape are largely due to the bizarre handling of Hitler's and Eva Braun's corpses that left far too many unanswered questions.

These strange circumstances deserve review to arrive at the most credible findings from the autopsy reports, the likely modes of death for Hitler and Braun, and to determine if the body autopsied was that of Adolf Hitler.

THE FORENSIC PATHOLOGY OF ADOLF HITLER

Morris Leikind wrote a report for the American intelligence community in 1945, but it was not declassified until 2000. The report incorrectly held that the two burned bodies in the garden of the Chancellery were never discovered by the Soviets. At the conclusion of the war, the American military had no clear understanding as to what the Soviets had found or that the burned bodies had been subjected to forensic examination.

In accordance with the Nazi Crimes Disclosure Act, the Central Intelligence Agency in the year 2000 released the declassified autopsy report of Adolf Hitler. It was learned that soon after overrunning the *Führerbunker* at the base of the Chancellery, the Soviet Red Army exhumed two partially burned bodies. A seven-member team of Soviet forensic pathologists examined the presumed remains of Hitler and Braun. Lev A. Bezymenski, a Soviet journalist and interpreter, generated a report describing the forensic findings. As an aside Bezymenski later became a Soviet historian and conduit for Soviet propaganda. Joseph Stalin took great interest in the autopsy and influenced the subsequent report by Bezymenski.

The autopsy described the corpse of a man greatly disfigured by fire. The body was deemed between the ages of fifty and sixty years (Hitler was fifty-six when he died). The height measured 165 centimeters, but the measurements were approximate due to the charring of the flesh. Converting 165 centimeters to feet and inches arrives at almost five feet five inches. Hitler's medical and military records listed him at five feet eight inches, a discrepancy possibly resulting from the charring of the flesh and/or stooping of his pre-morbid posture.

Parts of the occipital bone and the left temporal bone were present along with cheekbones and nasal bones. The report stated that the charred tongue had its tip firmly locked between the teeth of the upper and lower jaws. Examination of the upper jaw found nine teeth connected by a gold bridge. Pins on the second left and the second right incisor anchored the bridge. This dental work proved highly distinctive and, as we shall see, provides the strongest evidence that the body autopsied was that of Adolf Hitler.

The two most surprising and suspicious aspects of Lev Bezymenski's report consisted of his claim that splinters of glass and parts of a thin-walled ampoule were located within the mouth of the male cadaver. This spoke to a broken ampoule of poison (cyanide). A second unusual feature was reportedly found when examining Hitler's genitalia. The report documented only one testicle within the singed scrotum, that being the right one. The left testicle could not be located either in the scrotum or within the inguinal canal.

After the fall of the Soviet Union many years later, it came to light that Stalin had wished Hitler an ignoble death and ordered his death be reported as caused by poisoning. Stalin did not wish Hitler the heroic or manly death of a self-inflicted gunshot wound. Dying from poisoning was generally viewed as the death of a coward. Bezymenski in 1968 published *The Death of Adolf Hitler* and admitted in his book that the original report contained many deliberate lies, such as Hitler dying of poisoning.

Bezymenski and the forensic pathologists knew of Stalin's desire to paint Hitler in the worst possible light, and fearing for their lives, wisely accommodated the Soviet dictator's wishes. The report of the single right testicle also smacks of being bogus. In *The Secret Diaries of Hitler's Doctor* Dr. Morell's notes described Hitler's cremasteric reflexes as being intact. Morell's description of intact cremasteric reflexes requires the presence of *two* testicles. This clinical finding alone negates the autopsy's findings.

The cremasteric reflex is elicited by stroking the inner, upper aspect of the male thigh with a slow and light scrape of a pin and is interpreted by observing the simultaneous retraction of the testicle on that side. Morell's examination revealed Hitler's cremasteric reflexes to be intact, indicating *two* testicles with normal retraction of both. This finding has not previously been reported to this author's knowledge but has been hidden in plain sight ever since the discovery of Morell's medical casebook of Hitler, titled by Irving *The Secret Diaries of Hitler's Doctor*.

Nevertheless, it is also worth recalling the rumormongering among the Allied soldiers, and the derogatory ditty, claiming Hitler had but one ball (see chapter 9). Perhaps the forensic report included this attention-getting tidbit to bolster earlier rumors and to further deprecate Hitler's manliness.

Over-reactive cremasteric reflexes may be present in youth. When this over-reactive response occurs, the testicle may withdraw so far back that an examiner might incorrectly determine that the testicle did not lie within the scrotal sac.

It is possible, but unlikely, that the rumor of Hitler having only one testicle might have come from his childhood doctor. This is at least a possibility, though it seems unlikely given that general physicians do not usually attempt to elicit cremasteric reflexes in youthful healthy boys. The Nazis confiscated and destroyed Dr. Bloch's medical records, and none are available to provide clarification.

Another unusual finding, as noted earlier, was the tongue tightly clenched between his upper and lower jaws. This finding suggests terminal convulsions (a generalized seizure), and indeed convulsions can occur with cyanide poisoning. However, this finding is suspicious and may have been purposely inserted into the report to mislead and enhance the false notion of cyanide poisoning. A conclusion on this description cannot be determined with certainty, but more likely than not, the finding of Hitler's tongue clenched between his jaws is bogus.

SOURCES OF CONFUSION RELATING TO HITLER'S DEATH

Joseph Stalin privately accepted the forensic findings relating to Adolf Hitler, but nevertheless embroidered suspicion in public and especially among the Western Allies. Despite Stalin's belief that Hitler had died in the bunker, he sought to mislead the Western Allies on this matter. Stalin claimed Hitler might have escaped at the last minute from a besieged Berlin and lived on in Spain or South America. He also demanded that Gen. Georgy Zhukov misinform the press by claiming it was possible that Hitler had escaped by plane from Berlin.

Why Stalin sowed confusion by hiding information learned when the Red Army overran Hitler's bunker is unclear but may relate to his wanting to prompt an expensive and fruitless search for Hitler by the Western intelligence services. Stalin also went on to suggest that the Western Allies might have hidden Hitler, furthering his wishes to disparage his former allies as traitorous in the eyes of the world.

In any event Stalin's conspiratorial machinations spawned multiple "sightings" of Hitler throughout the world and gave rise to a flurry of poorly documented claims. As recently as 2011, the book *Grey Wolf: The Escape of Adolf Hitler* by Simon Dunstan and Gerrard Williams claimed that Hitler and Braun did not commit suicide but instead escaped Germany and traveled to South America by way of a German U-boat. Historians have dismissed this book's thesis. The highly respected British historian Guy Walters went even further by referring to their claim as "rubbish."

None of the conspiracy theories refute the compelling evidence presented by Hitler's unique dental work, nor do they invalidate the testimonials of those who lived in the bunker with Hitler. The conspiracy theories also fail to address how

Hitler might have survived for any significant amount of time, given his serious heart and neurological diseases. Both his major illnesses were life-shortening and occurred before effective treatments came into existence. Nevertheless, such conspiracy theories continue to draw attention especially on late night cable television and in periodicals with limited journalistic ethics.

Lavrenti Beria, head of the NKVD (People's Commissariat for Internal Affairs of the Soviet Union), initiated "Operation Myth," wishing to discredit his rivals in SMERSH, an umbrella organization consisting of three counter-intelligence organizations within the Red Army. Beria's NKVD failed to share evidence that Hitler had died of a gunshot wound to the head. The operation to gather such evidence involved harsh interrogations of the captive occupants of the bunker. These prisoners were subjected to long imprisonments. This closely held information was reported to Stalin but otherwise kept secret from the world until well after Stalin's death.

Troops of the Soviet Third Army carried the presumed corpses of Hitler and Braun along with them when leaving Berlin. In early June 1945, the Soviets reburied the autopsied bodies in a forest near the town of Rathenau, Germany. Eight months later they dug them up again and moved the remains to the more secure Soviet army's garrison in Magdeburg located about a hundred miles by car from Berlin. In 1970 the Soviets decided to abandon the garrison and return it to the East German civilian authorities.

According to a CNN report datelined "Moscow December 11, 2009," the Soviets belatedly reported they had burned the Hitler remains so that the site at Magdeburg might never become a memorial to fascism or Nazi ideals. Yuri Andropov, secretary of the Central Committee of the USSR at the time, made the final decision. According to the CNN article, Vasily Khristoforov, the head archivist of Russia's Federal Security Services (successor to the KGB), reported the bodies had been burned in 1970 and that the ashes had been dumped into a river. Fragments of the skull and the jawbone, the only remaining material from the autopsy, had been transferred and securely stored for many years in the State Archives in Moscow.

HOW TO MAKE SENSE OF IT ALL

Newspaper articles in the *Independent*, *New York Times*, and *London Sunday Times* in 2013 describe the witness report of Rochus Misch, Hitler's last surviving bodyguard. Misch worked in the bunker and manned the telephone exchange. He recalled when Gen. Wilhelm Keitel reported that the German Army had failed to break the Soviet encirclement of Berlin, and that the end of the Second World War was inevitable. This final message from Keitel set in motion Hitler's suicide.

Rochus Misch described how the *Führer*, who was painfully aware of the humiliation visited upon Mussolini's corpse on April 28, 1945, directed his adjutant Otto Günsche that following his suicide Günsche was to burn his body. Misch's report is consistent with what Albert Speer shared in his memoir about Hitler's fear of humiliation as had been visited upon Mussolini's corpse only a few days earlier. Speer also added how Eva Braun had wished to die with Hitler in the bunker. Speer described how Hitler had chosen not to attempt an escape from Berlin, but rather die in Berlin along with its defenders. Misch saw Hitler speak to Martin Bormann just prior to entering his private quarters with Eva Braun. When the door had been closed to the private quarters, Günsche with an air of finality ordered no one to disturb Hitler, providing Hitler and Eva Braun their uninterrupted opportunity to commit suicide.

After some time had passed, a stirring occurred of those huddled outside Hitler's private quarters. Misch approached the then-open door and peeked inside. There he viewed Braun and Hitler lying dead on the couch. Eva sat to Hitler's left and had her legs curled up. Hitler sat near her, eyes open and staring, his head pitched slightly forward. His pistol lay nearby. Several others including Günsche and Hitler's valet, Linge, witnessed and confirmed the deaths of Hitler and Braun. Misch described seeing Hitler's body wrapped in a rug and carried out. Misch said he recognized Hitler's shoes that were visible from the end of the rolled carpet.

Only a small group of Nazis were present in the bunker at the time. Among these people were the new Chancellor Joseph Goebbels and Hitler's private secretary Martin Bormann, who would either commit suicide or else be killed within a matter of a few days. This greatly reduced the number of surviving witnesses to Hitler's death and along with the bogus Soviet reports provided ample room for the seeds of conspiracy to germinate and grow.

Misch related how Hitler had directed that following his death those who had served him in the bunker were released from any further service to the Third Reich. In accordance with this directive and after seeing Hitler dead, Misch tried to make his escape. His flight proved unsuccessful, and the Soviet Red Army soon captured him in Berlin. He was interviewed, tortured, and for the next eight years imprisoned in Soviet labor camps. After his long imprisonment Misch eventually made his way back to his native Berlin. There he was known to show up and give impromptu lectures at the site of the Führer's bunker and regularly share stories about the man he called "the boss."

Reports by people who were in the bunker with Hitler are persuasive but not altogether satisfying. For example, Rochus Misch remained unrepentant about his service to Hitler. He held that Hitler was a good boss and described Hitler's behavior in no way that would characterize him suffering from strange mental disorders. Could such reports as given by Misch be a final act of loyalty toward a favored boss and be designed to purposely mislead? This is possible, but the reports of Misch and others from the bunker have a ring of authenticity about them. Nevertheless, the reports in no way undermine evidence of the subtler neuropsychological changes that occur with advanced Parkinson's disease, nor do they alter reports of Hitler's well-known personality traits.

An article in *The World* by Jean-Marie Pottier dated April 30, 2018, describes skull fragments stored in the Russian State Archive. Following the fall of the Soviet Union, the staff members of the Archive were anxious to demonstrate more openness than its predecessors. Two investigative journalists, a Frenchman named Jean-Christophe Brisard and the Russian American Lana Parshina, along with help from Philippe Charlier, a French scientist, examined the remaining bone fragments said to be Hitler's. Charlier stated convincingly that the jawbone with its characteristic dental work was that of Adolf Hitler. He analyzed the teeth with a stereomicroscope and avowed that the jawbone presented to him was not a "historical forgery." He found correspondence between the jawbone with its dental work and the earlier radiographs taken by Hitler's dentist. Such evidence argues convincingly that Hitler died in Berlin and not in South America, Japan, Antarctica, or elsewhere.

Earlier reports on Hitler's highly characteristic dental work had been based on reports given by Käthe Heusermann, who was the dental assistant to Hitler's dentist. She confirmed that the extensive dental work and bridge was indeed that of Hitler. Hitler's dentist, Hugo Blaschke, also confirmed that he had performed the dental work found on the jawbone and identified it as that of Adolf Hitler. Similarly, Fritz Echtman, a dental technician involved in Hitler's care, also confirmed the jawbone with its dental work was that of Adolf Hitler. The identification was proven within a reasonable doubt and confirms the death of Adolf Hitler.

The skull said to be that of Hitler from the Soviet archives has been called into question. Based on DNA evidence it was determined to be that of a woman and estimated to have been the skull of a woman of less than forty years of age. Given the vast number of deaths in Berlin at that time, and the abundance of available corpses, this should not prove too surprising. The question arises, assuming the body of Braun was buried with Hitler's in the shallow grave, was it her skull? No proof exists that this was the skull of Eva Braun, but this remains a strong possibility. Clearly the skull was not that of Adolf Hitler.

The obvious discrepancy between the jawbone findings, for which strong evidence exists that it was that of Hitler, and equally strong evidence that it was not Hitler's skull bone creates consternation. The skull fragment with a bullet hole and shown to be that of a woman had been stored in a floppy disc storage box in the State Archive according to Jean-Marie Pottier. On the other hand, the jawbone had been stored in a cigarillo box in the FSB (Russia's Federal Security Service) archives, again according to Pottier. The two pieces of evidence had been handled differently and stored in different archives, and certainly such handling creates doubt as to whether they were related.

Regrettably the jawbone was never analyzed for DNA evidence. This is unfortunate, as such an investigation would have been helpful and potentially confirmatory. The fact that the Soviet government in 1970 destroyed all vestiges of Hitler's skeleton prevents any further DNA analysis from being performed.

In summary, Hitler's initial autopsy reports for starkly political reasons were distorted regarding his mode of death, were disparaging of Hitler's masculinity, and were made to conform to existing Soviet propaganda. Ultimately when the truth came out following the dissolution of the Soviet Union, the reports of Eva Braun dying from cyanide and Hitler dying from a self-inflicted gunshot wound to the head have been confirmed.

Nevertheless, the Soviet approach of forcing science to imitate official doctrine and its propaganda, as exemplified by the thoroughly debunked Lysenko era,* had a long and successful run within the former Soviet Union. Therein lies a compelling lesson in support for maintaining scientific integrity.

---

*Lysenkoism, named after the Soviet biologist Trofim Lysenko, claimed that crops changed based on environmental factors and thus are inheritable. Lysenkoism was applied to agriculture during the Stalin era with disastrous consequences leading to mass starvation.

CHAPTER 23

FINAL THOUGHTS REGARDING HITLER'S CULPABILITY

D id the impact of Hitler's abnormal physical and mental health mitigate his crimes against humanity? Understanding that Hitler in his later years was ill inevitably prompts this important question as to whether the Holocaust and the dastardly acts of the *Einsatzgruppen* on the Eastern Front should be viewed less judgmentally due to his poor health. The answer to these questions is a resounding NO!

Many historians have been scrupulous to avoid any reliance on behavioral and medical determinants simply because of their concerns for potentially being seen to reduce Hitler's personal responsibility. To be sure, the implications to this question have concerned many historians, behaviorists, journalists, and physicians. Various authors have tried to explain how such crimes against humanity could have come from an advanced and civilized society, as was Germany, and have wished not to diminish the blame that history has squarely placed upon Adolf Hitler and his followers.

Hans-Joachim Neumann and Henrik Eberle in their book *Was Hitler Ill?* laid out Hitler's diseases and described his slow physical and mental decline. But the authors then go to the extreme by inexplicably claiming, "There is no evidence that these two conditions [age-related arteriosclerosis and Parkinson's disease] affected his decisions." Neumann and Eberle conclude by saying that Hitler "was healthy and accountable."

Yes, Hitler was accountable for his actions, but he was *not* healthy. The fact that he was unhealthy does not mitigate his crimes against humanity. Neumann and Eberle, one trained as a dentist and the other as a historian, appear unaware that cognitive changes occur in advanced Parkinson's disease and that these cognitive changes can fall well short of dementia. A lack of appreciation of this clinical aspect of Parkinson's disease may result either from an abundance of caution to even hint at mitigation of Hitler's (and by extension German society's) responsibilities for crimes against humanity, or an unawareness of this neuropsychological feature with advanced Parkinson's disease. Likewise, Hitler's hypertensive cardiovascular disease and coronary artery disease had serious implications for his life expectancy. Certainly, Hitler was *not* a healthy man.

In the popular media a tendency exists today to reduce *der Führer* to a simplistic caricature. Oftentimes he is described as mad or crazy, but such oversimplifications miss the flesh and blood complexity of the man. Hitler was not psychotic. He was not *non compos mentis*. He was not clinically insane.

No evidence exists of Hitler suffering a major psychosis such as schizophrenia or bipolar disorder. Nor was he demented. Hitler was clearly intelligent and capable as demonstrated by his meteoric rise to becoming chancellor of Germany. He possessed highly unusual personality traits even as a young man and was both a loner and a misfit. Nevertheless, his unusual personality traits proved enormously alluring for desperate Germans and attracted throngs of fawning admirers. Such political success and adulation are often seen with individuals who demonstrate grandiose narcissism as did Hitler.

Hitler's charismatic behavior shown forth at a time when such grandiosity and radicalism appealed to desperate, war-weary, and recession-suffering Germans who longed for overly simplistic answers and an easy scapegoat to blame for their discomfort. After all, post–World War I Germany politically was a boiling cauldron, steeped in revolutionary zeal, suffering from national disgrace and humiliation, and brimming with utter indignation. The German nation proved ripe for a demagogue who campaigned on the promise to "Make Germany Great Again."

Adolf Hitler's medical issues cannot and should not be used to diminish his cruelty, destructive nature, and genocidal behavior. During only the last years of his life, Parkinson's disease reduced his response speed and ability to comprehend and reply to disparate streams of information in a timely fashion. His neurological disease did not give rise to Hitler's virulent anti-Semitism, megalomania, and brutality toward others—all personality characteristics formed well prior to the onset of his Parkinson's disease.

While Hitler had suffered from lifelong intestinal disturbances, his more major illnesses of Parkinson's disease and coronary artery disease did not appear until he was well into his forties. Each of these major chronic and life-shortening illnesses individually reduced his predicted life expectancy to about eight years from onset, and even more so in combination, and are believed to have been factors in hastening his timeframe for securing *Lebensraum*, Aryan domination, and destruction of the Jewish/Bolshevik state.

His chronic Parkinson's disease also impaired his mental flexibility and created a mental stickiness that slowed transitioning from one concept to the next. This mild frontal lobe dysfunction reduced his ability to quickly make military decisions and by so doing impaired the performance of Germany's military.

While not life-shortening, Hitler's acute illnesses in August and September 1941 were likely a bacteria-related enteritis (dysentery) followed by a severe gall bladder attack and struck at a critical time during the initial phases of Operation Barbarossa. Hitler's prostration at this propitious time allowed his generals to include their goal of capturing Moscow in addition to Hitler's original plans for Operation Barbarossa, that being to capture Leningrad in the north and in the south the Ukraine breadbasket and the Caucasus oil fields. The overextension of the German forces that the addition of Moscow required doomed to defeat an already risky German military operation.

Hitler, as the supreme German leader, maintained tight control over the government, security forces, and military. His well-documented control needs, particularly evident during the latter phases of the war, limited his attempt to distance himself from the genocide in the concentration camps and the cruelty of the *Einsatzgruppen* on the Eastern Front. Hitler was careful not to leave orders signed by him that incriminated him in the Holocaust. Nevertheless, his involvement and inspiration for genocide and the cruelty of the *Einsatzgruppen* simply cannot be denied. In short, Hitler, while unhealthy, was fully accountable and cognizant of his actions. Hitler is due no mitigation of his culpability for the death and destruction that he inflicted upon the world.

Hitler's extreme grandiosity, stubbornness, mental inflexibility, and obsessive hatred of non-Aryans, especially Jews and Slavs, along with his obsession for *Lebensraum* led to the wartime devastation of Europe. As for Adolf Hitler's poor health late in his life and his lifelong personality flaws, they eventually reduced his overall effectiveness for reaching his long-term political and military goals. These features intrinsic to Adolf Hitler, along with other extrinsic historical, political, and economic factors, became the prescription for Nazi Germany's defeat in World War II.

FURTHER READING

Ambrose, Stephen E. *D-Day: What Hitler Did Wrong*. World War II History, info, converted from *D-Day: June 6, 1944: The Climactic Battle of World War II*. New York: Simon and Schuster, 1995.

Attkisson, Sharyl. *The Smear: How Shady Political Operatives and Fake News Control What You See, What You Think, and How You Vote*. New York: Harper Collins, 2017.

Bezymenski, Lev A. *The Death of Adolf Hitler: Unknown Documents from Soviet Archives*. Released by the Central Intelligence Agency according to the Nazi War Crimes Disclosure Act, 2001 and 2007. New York: Harcourt, Brace and World, 1968.

Binion, Rudolph. *Hitler among the Germans*. DeKalb: Northern Illinois University Press, 1976.

Bloch, Eduard, as told by J. D. Ratcliff. *"My Patient, Hitler": A Memoir of Hitler's Jewish Physician*. Originally in two parts, in March 15 and March 22, 1941, issues of *Collier's* magazine. Later in *Journal for Historical Review* 14, no. 3 (May–June 1994): 27–35.

Brain, Lord Russell, and John N. Walton. *Brain's Diseases of the Nervous System*. New York: Oxford University Press, 1969.

Breo, Dennis L. *Hitler's Medical File*. American Medical Association from American Medical News, in *Chicago Tribune*, October 14, 1985.

Bromberg, Norbert, and Verna Small. *Hitler's Psychopathology*. New York: International Universities Press, 1983.

Campbell, John. *Naval Weapons of World War Two*. New York: Conway Maritime Press, 1985.

Churchill, Winston S. *Triumph and Tragedy*. Boston: Houghton Mifflin, 1953.

Dunstan, Simon, and Gerrard Williams. *Grey Wolf: The Escape of Adolf Hitler*. New York: Sterling, 2011.

Fest, Joaquin. *Hitler*. New York: Harcourt Brace, 1974.

Feuchtwanger, Edgar. *Hitler, My Neighbor: Memories of a Jewish Childhood*. New York: Other Press, 2013.

Fox, Margalit. "Rochus Misch, Bodyguard of Hitler, Dies at 96." *New York Times*, September 7, 2013.

Friedman, George. "This Map Shows Germany's Critical Mistakes Fighting Russia in WWII." Editorial in *Mauldin Economics*, November 29, 2017.

Fritz, Stephen G. *The First Soldier: Hitler As Military Leader*. New Haven, CT: Yale University Press, 2018.

Frost, Natasha. *Hitler's Teeth Reveal Nazi Dictator's Cause of Death*. History Stories, May 19, 2018.

Gompert, David C. "Binnendijk, Hans, and Lin, Bonny. Hitler's Decision to Invade the USSR 1941." In *Blinders, Blunders, and War*. Rand Corporation, 2014.

Goñi, Uki. "Tests on Skull Fragment Cast Doubt on Adolf Hitler Suicide Story." *The Guardian*, September 26, 2009.

Gorlitz, Walter, ed. *The Memoirs of Field Marshal Wilhelm Keitel, Chief of the German High Command 1938–1945*. Translated by David Irving. New York: Cooper Square Press, 2000.

Guderian, Heinz. *Achtung Panzer! The Development of Tank Warfare*. First published in 1937. English language version London: Orion Books, 1992.

Haffner, Sebastian. *Defying Hitler: A Memoir*. New York: Farrar, Straus, and Giroux, 2000.

Hamann, Brigitte. *Hitler's Vienna: A Dictator's Apprenticeship*. New York: Oxford University Press, 1999.

Hayden, Deborah. *Pox: Genius, Madness, and the Mysteries of Syphilis*. New York: Basic Books, 2003.

Heston, Leonard L., and Renate Heston. *Adolf Hitler: A Medical Descent That Changed History, His Drug Abuse, Doctors, and Illnesses*. Portland, OR: Baypoint Publishers, 1999.

———. *The Medical Casebook of Adolf Hitler*. London: William Kimber, 1979.

History.com. "The Battle of the Bulge." October 14, 2009.

Hitler, Paula. "My Brother the *Führer*." In Blogging World War Two. October 28, 2016.

Hoehn, M. M., and M. D. Yahr. "Parkinsonism: Onset Progression and Mortality." *Neurology* 17 (2006): 427–44.

Hutton, J. T., and J. L. Morris. "Adolph Hitler's Parkinsonism May Have Influenced the Battle of Normandy and the Outcome of World War II." Parkinsonism and Related Disorders, Abstracts of the XIII International Congress on Parkinson's Disease, July 24–28, 1999, Vancouver, Canada, S119.

Hutton, Tom. *Carrying the Black Bag: A Neurologist's Bedside Tales*. Lubbock:

Texas Tech University Press, 2015.

Interrogation II with Paula Hitler. National Archives and Records Administration, Textual Archives Service Section.

Interview with Paula Wolf. Eisenhower Library website, National Archives and Records Administration.

Irving, David. *The Secret Diaries of Hitler's Doctor.* New York: Macmillan Publishing, 1983.

Jetzinger, Franz. *Hitler's Youth.* London: Hutchinson, 1958.

Keitel, Wilhelm. *The Memoirs of Field-Marshal Wilhelm Keitel: Chief of the German Command, 1938–1945.* New York: Cooper Square Press, 2000.

Kershaw, Ian. *Hitler: A Biography.* New York: W. W. Norton, 1998.

Kubizek, August. *The Young Hitler I Knew: The Definitive Inside Look at the Artist Who Became a Monster.* Yorkshire: Frontline Books, 2011.

Langer, Walter C. *The Mind of Adolf Hitler: The Secret Wartime Report.* New York: Basic Books, 1972.

Langston, J. W., P. A. Ballard, J. W. Tetrud, and I. Irwin. "Chronic Parkinsonism in Humans Due to a Product of Meperidine-Analog Synthesis." *Science* 219 (1983): 979–80.

Leikind, Morris. "Studies in Pathography, Adolph Hitler." Released as result of Nazi War Crimes Disclosure Act 2000. CIA Special Collections Release in full, 2000.

Lieberman, Abraham. "Historical Brief: Hitler's Parkinson's Disease Began in 1933." *Movement Disorders* 12, no. 2 (1997): 239–40.

Martin, Sharon. "Adult Children of Alcoholics and the Need to Feel in Control." Blog. Happily Imperfect for Psych Central.com, December 29, 2017.

Maser, Werner. *Hitler: Legend, Myth, and Reality.* New York: Harper & Row, 1973, translated from the German, *Hitler: Legende, Mythos und Realität,* Munich, 1971.

Meyer, Nigel. *Battle of the Bulge: Ardennes Offensive Article.* Military History Tours. August 31, 2015.

Miller, Alice. *For Your Own Good: Hidden Cruelty in Child-Rearing and the Roots of Violence.* New York: Farrar, Straus, and Giroux, 1980.

Misch, Rochus. "Adolf Hitler's 'Last Bodyguard' Reveals What Happened in Nazi Leader's Final Minutes in the Berlin Bunker." *Independent,* March 22, 2013.

Miss Cellania, "Der Fartenführer: The Story of Hitler's Illnesses." *Uncle John's Endlessly Engrossing Bathroom Reader.* Monday, March 24, 2014.

Neumann, Hans-Joachim, and Henrik Eberle. *Was Hitler Ill?* Malden, MA: Polity

Press, 2013.

Ohler, Norman. *Blitzed*. New York: Houghton Mifflin Harcourt, 2017.

O'Reilly, Bill. *Hitler's Last Days: The Death of the Nazi Regime and the World's Most Notorious Dictator*. New York: Henry Holt, 2015.

Orlow, Dietrich. Review of *Totalitarian Politics and Sexual Perversion: The Case of Adolf Hitler* by Robert G. L. Waite. *Journal of Interdisciplinary History* IX, no. 3 (Winter 1979): 500–515.

Parkinson, J. *An Essay on the Shaking Palsy*. London: Sherwood, Neely and Jones, 1817.

Patterson, Tony. "Hitler Was Ordered to Trim His Mustache." *Telegraph*, May 6, 2007.

Pottier, Jean-Marie. "They Saved Hitler's Skull. Or Did They?" *In the World*, April 30, 2018.

Redlich, Fritz. *Hitler: Diagnosis of a Destructive Prophet*. New York: Oxford University Press, 1999.

Sandberg, D. E., H. F. Meyer-Behlburg, G. S. Aranoff, J. M. Sconzo, and T. W. Hensle. "Boys with Hypospadias: A Survey of Behavioral Difficulties." *J. Pediatr Psychol* 14 no. 4 (December 1989): 491–514.

Showell, Jak. *Hitler's Navy: A Reference Guide to the Kriegsmarine 1935–1945*. Barnsley, UK: Seaforth Publishing, 2009.

Sognnaes, Reidar F., and Ferdinant Strom. "The Odontological Identification of Adolf Hitler: Definitive Documentation by X-rays, Interrogations and Autopsy Findings." *Acta Odontologica Scandinavica* 31, no. 1 (1973).

Soukup, V., and R. L. Adams. "Parkinson's Disease." In *Neuropsychology for Clinical Practice*, edited by R. L. Adams, O. A. Parsons, J. L. Culbertson, et al., 243–67. Washington, DC: American Psychological Association, 1997.

Speer, Albert. "Foreword." In *The Medical Casebook of Adolf Hitler*, Leonard L. Heston and Renate Heston. London: William Kimber, 1979.

———. *Inside the Third Reich: Memoirs by Albert Speer*. New York: Simon & Schuster, 1970.

Stahel, David. *Operation Barbarossa and Germany's Defeat in the East*. New York: Cambridge University Press, 2009.

Stierlin, Helm. *Adolf Hitler: A Family Perspective*. New York: The Psychohistory Press, 1976.

Tkachenko, Maxim. "Official: KGB Chief Ordered Hitler's Remains Destroyed." CNN, December 11, 2009.

Toland, John. *Adolf Hitler*, Vol. 1. New York: Doubleday, 1976.

———. *Adolf Hitler*, Vol. 2. New York: Doubleday, 1976.

Trevor-Roper, H. R. *The Last Days of Hitler*, 3rd ed. New York: Collier Books, 1962.

Trueheart, Charles. "Who Killed Hitler's Niece, Reconsidered." *The Washington Post*, 1992.

Ullrich, Volker. *Hitler: Ascent, 1889–1939*. New York: Vintage Books, 2017.

———. *Hitler: Downfall, 1939–1945*. New York: Alfred A. Knopf, 2020.

Waite, Robert G. L. *The Psychopathic God Adolf Hitler*. New York: Basic Books, 1977.

Warfare History Network. The Center for National Interest. "Hitler's 5 'Wonder' Weapons of World War II," 2020.

Weber, Thomas. *Becoming Hitler: The Making of a Nazi*. New York: Basic Books, 2017.

———. *Hitler's First War: Adolf Hitler, The Men of the List Regiment*. Oxford University Press, 2011.

Wilson, James M. Personal communication.

Woilitz, Janet G. *Adult Children of Alcoholics*. Deerfield Beach, FL: Health Communications, Inc. 1983.

INDEX

Note: Page numbers in *italics* refer to illustrations.

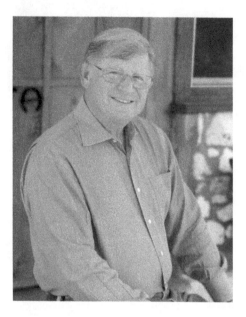

Tom Hutton, MD, PhD, is an internationally recognized clinical and research neurologist and educator. The past president of the Texas Neurological Society, Dr. Hutton served as professor and vice chairman of the Department of Medical and Surgical Neurology at the Texas Tech School of Medicine. He now lives on his cattle ranch near Fredericksburg, Texas.

Printed in the USA
CPSIA information can be obtained
at www.ICGtesting.com
LVHW092242010224
770720LV00006B/155